MORE THAN I AM

Celebrating
30 Years of Publishing
in India

MORE THAN I AM

YOGA WISDOM
for 21st century teens

Varuna Shunglu
and Ken Spillman

PHOTOGRAPHS
Kanishk Gupta, Rohan Chakravarty

ILLUSTRATIONS
Suvidha Mistry

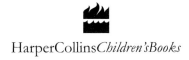

HarperCollins*Children'sBooks*

First published in India in 2023 by HarperCollins Children's Books
An imprint of HarperCollins *Publishers*
Building No. 10, Tower A, 4th Floor, DLF Cyber City, Phase II, Gurugram, 122002, India
www.harpercollins.co.in

2 4 6 8 10 9 7 5 3 1

Text © Varuna Shunglu and Ken Spillman 2023
Illustrations © HarperCollins *Publishers* India 2023

P-ISBN: 978-93-5629-483-7
E-ISBN: 978-93-5629-484-4

Typeset and designed in Sabon 11 pt/16 pt
by Veena, Bookwatch

Printed and bound at Nutech Print Services - India

Contents

Foreword by Bhanumathi Narasimhan 7

1. Why Yoga 9

2. The Present Moment 15

3. The Concept of Energy 23

4. Mental Machinery 31

5. Daily Practices to Boost Energy 47

6. The Budding You 63

7. Believing in Balance 77

8. Loving the Cosmic You! 89

   21-day Sankalpa 95

   Glossary 104

   Further Reading 106

Foreword

Yoga comes from the root word 'yuj' meaning union. But what is the union? Gurudev Sri Sri Ravi Shankar says it is the wave uniting with its depth. The union with the Self; when the small 'i' dissolves in the big 'I'; when the individual soul merges with the infinite boundless consciousness. Your state at that time is called yoga.

The physical postures are one aspect of ashtanga yoga and culminate in meditation leading to samadhi. This is the way forward. Every step is the preparation for samadhi; preparing the body to hold the light or the energy that comes out of samadhi. When both body and mind are in harmony then samadhi happens, in equilibrium, and that is when a person is called a yogi. Till then you are doing yoga. Becoming a yogi means one who gets the ability to be in the self.

This book, written by dear Varuna with Ken Spillman, is entitled *More Than I Am*. It is a very interesting title and is also apt because yoga is more than the small 'i' which keeps saying, 'I am the body'. It is the expanded awareness, the undivided unified consciousness, the infinite field of possibilities.

Varuna is a sincere girl with depth, on a wonderful journey as a writer. I love books, and enjoying reading is a quality of consciousness that makes you steadfast, stable and focused. In fact, when you start reading books with such depth, you can read between the lines too and it takes you to the right path.

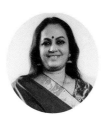

BHANUMATHI NARASIMHAN
Chair, Women's Welfare and Child Care
The Art of Living
AUTHOR: *Gurudev: On the Plateau of the Peak*, Westland Publications;
Sita: A Tale of Ancient Love, Penguin Books;
Gods and Goddesses, HarperCollins Children's Books

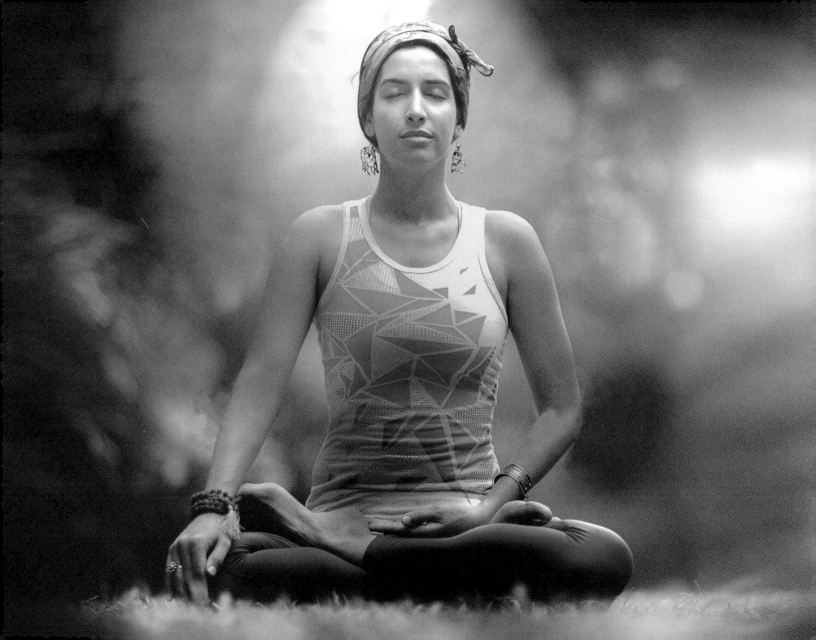

1
Why Yoga

The wisdom of yoga transforms one from craving for freedom to recognition of unboundedness, from limited ownership to oneness with the whole.

SRI SRI RAVI SHANKAR
spiritual leader and humanitarian

What does yoga really mean? More importantly, what can it mean for YOU?

Perhaps you've never given such questions more than a moment's thought. After all, who has time to ponder when we know all too well that the world will come to an end unless we somehow get that grade everyone's expecting? Or if we miss that movie? Or if that one person doesn't like our latest Instagram reel?

Isn't yoga just something that's supposed to be good for you, like vegetables, tuition and sport?

Well, yes, yoga IS good for you.

But here's the thing: yoga is good for you in more ways than you can possibly know. It has the power to make you more than you are – and more than you've ever imagined you could be.

> Yoga is a multipurpose life tool, ready to help you pass through the gateway to your best self – healthy, happy, strong and energetic, just as you want to be.

When you're growing up, it can often seem that there are too many questions and too few answers.

1. Who am I?
2. Why am I here?
3. Why do I need to do this?
4. Why aren't things easier?
5. What's the point?
6. How can I be strong?

It may be useful to think about yoga as a powerful search engine that can help us find the answers we are looking for.

Yoga does not simply mean an asana or three. It isn't standing on your head as your feet point to the heavens, and it isn't sitting silently for hours like a sage.

Google throws up many options to choose from when you type in a keyword. Similarly, yoga helps you sort through a huge amount of irrelevant information using a system of tried and tested codes. It unifies your mind, body and breath to help you get to the answers you need – and can make you joyful every day!

> **Y:** You are special
> **O:** One pointed focus
> **G:** Get ready to stretch your limits
> **A:** Always keep that smile

You are special

That is what yoga will tell you. We practise yoga to understand and recognize the roles we play in our lives – student, daughter, son, friend, etc. Above these roles lies a 'greater self', a special self that knows that we are MORE than all that we do in life. Yoga teaches us to discover ourselves every day.

One pointed focus

Is there an app that can 'boost' the speed of the mind? Or maybe 'erase' the junk from our heads that dances about in a loop? The practice of yoga can be your 'daily cleaner', sorting the trash and stress and throwing them out after a long hectic day at school. It not only clears and de-stresses the mind but also helps us

concentrate on the things that mean the world to us – our friends, family and study. It makes us more creative and agile when we play, work or have fun.

Awareness creates one pointed focus in our minds – to be kind, gentle, look after our environment, watch what we eat, live healthily and, most importantly, do something that makes a difference! Yoga brings this awareness in us.

Get ready to stretch your limits

Yoga can better equip us to face challenges in life.

> **A:** Awaken your mind
> **W:** Watchful
> **A:** Actively conscious
> **R:** Reach out
> **E:** Engage in positive thinking and action

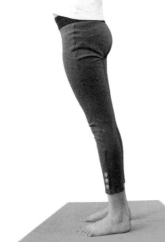

An imbalance in breath, it is said, can cause many imbalances in the body and lead to a lack of health. The correct pranayamas, asanas and meditation can strengthen not only the internal organs, tissues and bones but also steady the mind as we go from strength to strength.

Practising yoga and meditation every day can change the way we feel about ourselves and our goals as we find the cupboard that can lead us to our very own Narnia.

Always keep that smile

A smile is the greatest manifestation of a calm mind. Whenever we get stressed, the energy or prana in the body becomes low. All we need to do at these times is plug in our charger into the infinite electrical source that is the invisible universe around us.

The more we meditate, the larger the smile grows, the more our energies RISE!

MEDITATION = CALM + EFFORTLESS AWARENESS

IMPACT OF YOGA ON HEALTH AND DIGESTION: Eighteen teens with complaints of abdominal pain took a six-week yoga intervention* where 50 per cent felt an improvement in the pain, sleep and visceral sensitivity, that is, internal pain and discomfort.

* a study done under observation

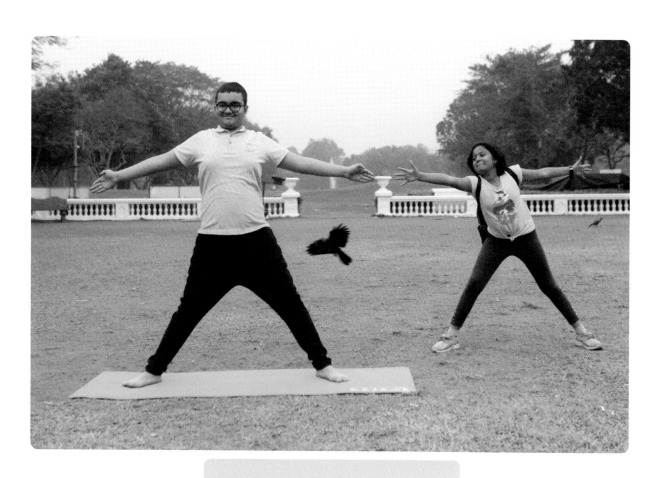

SMILE + STRETCH = YOGA EVERY DAY

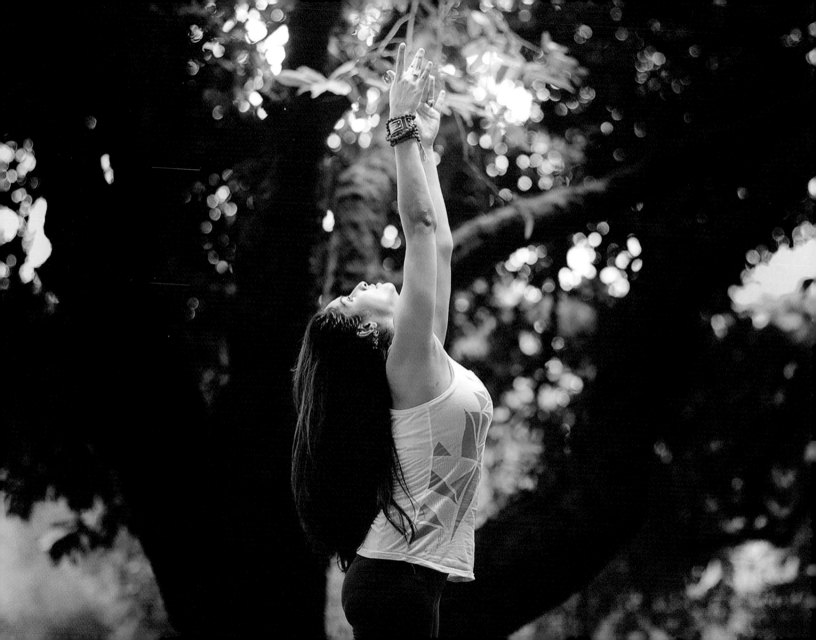

2

The Present Moment

Whatever the present moment contains, accept it as if you
had chosen it. Always work with it, not against it.

ECKHART TOLLE
author

All action can only happen in the present moment.

What is the present moment?

Each moment is the present moment.

Yes, it's easier said than done. It is a Herculean task to be in the present moment at ALL times but when we do certain things, our mind automatically comes back to the present moment.

There is No Other Way but to do it NOW!

Mind and our potential

Thousands of years have passed since sages and philosophers discovered the key to happiness – the key with the power to unlock our full potential.

There were two aspects to this. First, they spoke of the need to retrain oneself to stop regretting past actions and events. The second was retraining the mind to stop stressing about the future.

We only have to think for a moment to realize that we are bombarded by thoughts about the past or the future. Since no one can change the past or completely control the future, it was clear to the ancient sages that such thoughts were the source of all regret, sorrow, stress, fear and anxiety. *Yoga chitta vritti nirodha*, they said.

In essence, this means that dedicated practice over time makes it possible to control the inclination of the mind to attach itself to negative thoughts arising from our experience or beliefs about the past and our perceptions about the future.

P: Positive

R: Remain calm

E: Endeavour and strive (give your ALL to a task)

S: Send out goodness

E: Enable others

N: Never say never

T: Talk about ideas (creativity)

PRESENT = AWARENESS + POSITIVE ACTION

Such a practice involves uniting the mind, the body and the breath in the present moment – in other words, yoga.

When the mind is cleared of unnecessary thought, it becomes still.

It becomes focused like a laser beam attached only to the experience in the present moment.

In this state of clarity, we are capable of being fully aware, alert and sharp, observing all that is happening around us. We are able to see our troubles and stress as separate from ourselves. Without the stress of the world on our shoulders, we become playful. We become light and happy. When we start enjoying the present moment without sprinting into the past or future, we become masters of our minds.

If we really want to enjoy life to the fullest, we've got to do it in the present. Even if you don't like doing something that you need to do, do it with a smile. Have fun with it. Make the most of everything – even boring things. Then you will always enjoy yourself. This is an ancient rule of life.

TIME MANAGEMENT

I feel overwhelmed by the number of things I have to finish. My submissions, meeting my friends or even waking up on time feels difficult. I am always the last person to reach anywhere.

- Don't leave everything for the last moment. Always plan a day in advance. Keep your clothes out, do your homework on time.
- Resolutions last only if you convert them into habits. You will automatically put your things in their correct place, reach out for healthier food options and get ready to hit the sack at 10 p.m. instead of midnight.
- Make one small change every day starting with morning meditation.

So, how does being in the present help us tap into our undiscovered, unrealized and unlimited potential?

Potential is all the wonderful things we can be. It's just that we haven't fully discovered what they are yet. Potential is the difference between what you are and the best version of yourself.

Wouldn't you like to know what amazing things you are capable of? When Abraham Maslow said, 'What a man can be, he must be', he was talking about each person's need to be their best self, every moment of every day.

Cultivating habits

Have you heard your teacher say, 'This child has potential'?

It makes you wonder if there's some hidden treasure that you need to find. The truth is, potential is only the beginning of what you can achieve. You have some qualities and there are others that you discover along the way. The more qualities you cultivate, the more tools you have to excel. You may have realized quite early that you are good with numbers, talented in music or a strong runner.

The situations you are put into and the people you meet help uncover your potential. However, it is cultivating strong habits that will help you turn that hidden potential into something powerful. For example, you love coding on the computer. You and your parents cultivated that interest and you began learning more.

ACTIVITY: Write down one thing you're grateful for on a piece of paper. Fold the paper and put the chit in a glass/plastic jar. Do this every day. If you ever need a little hope, open one or more of those chits and read them.

You now practise it every day. You might very well be on your way to creating a new algorithm or a digital platform that can change the world in the near future. The scope is unlimited.

To discover our full range of potential, however, we need to take some initiative. If all we do is procrastinate, then we only go about in a loop. In the clarity of the present moment, decisions that affect our lives can be made through a calm and intuitive mind that aids our progress in the right direction.

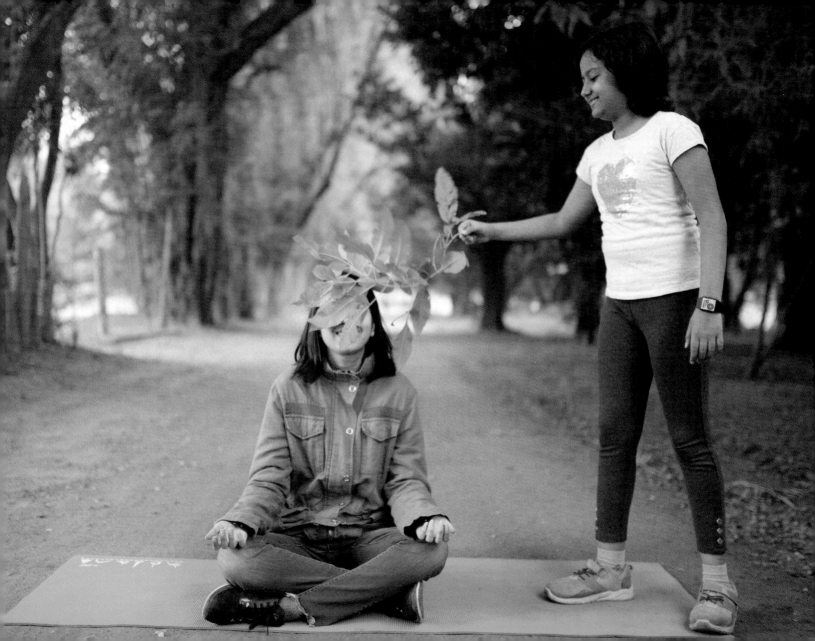

The ancients knew that positive action can only occur in the present moment. We can neither use a time machine to change what has already been done (or not done), nor leap into the future.

Imagine that you want to become a doctor. It would be pointless hoping for something in the future that magically hands you a career in medicine, right? In the present, however, you can take any number of actions that will help you to inch closer to your goal. You could study, talk to doctors, watch videos that show the process of getting into medical school or even read a book like this one to learn more about managing your life and maximizing your potential.

By creating small but impactful changes in our daily habits and patterns we can move towards our goals and empower ourselves.

Learning to surrender

At any point in time, we have choices about positive actions that might be taken. Sensible choices arise from clear thought in the present moment and the surrender of any thoughts that pull you away from your goal.

This power of surrender is never to be underestimated. It is the 'letting go' of negative forces within us that lightens the clutter in the mind. For example, you may surrender the anger within you – directed at a situation or person – so that it doesn't continue to bother you and so that you can carry on with whatever you need to do with a light and energetic mind.

Surrender can provide release and become an effective tool. Imagine you have a drone or model aircraft but keep holding on to it because you feel

DISCOVERING POTENTIAL = HARD WORK + POSITIVE ACTION + PLAYFULNESS + SURRENDER

afraid of it crashing. How would it fly? Once you have switched it on, you need to let go and watch the magic.

Next time you notice yourself holding on to negative thoughts, think of that drone.

Go fly.

Better than cold coffee in your study break!

GOOSEBERRY APPLE MOOD FIXER

INGREDIENTS
- gooseberry powder (amla powder) – 1/3 tsp
- jaggery/palm sugar – to taste
- green apple – one
- ginger, freshly grated
- water – half glass

HOW TO MAKE IT
Blend all the ingredients together in a mixer. Serve immediately.
This benefit-loaded, super healthy, delicious recipe increases immunity, boosts memory and satisfies that sugar craving!

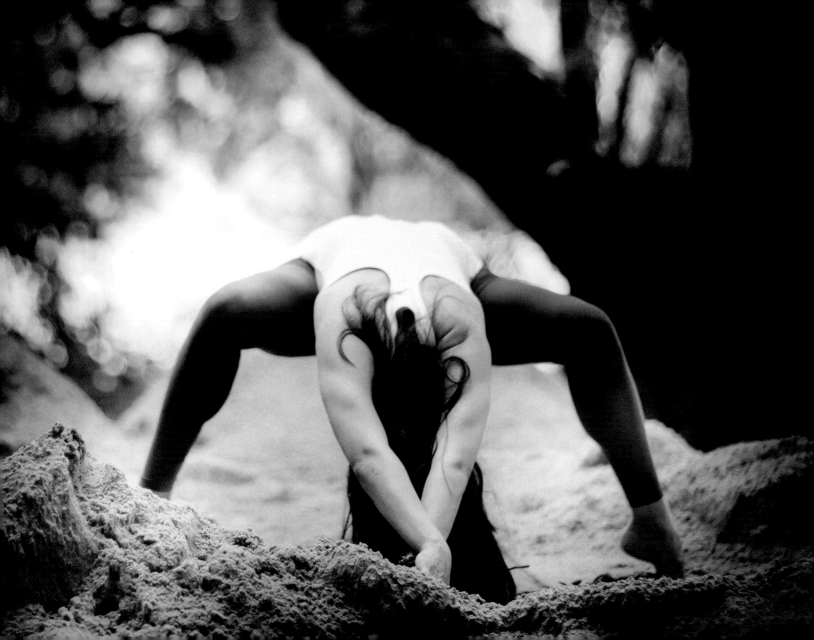

3

The Concept of Energy

*Sometimes I think the surest sign that intelligent life exists elsewhere
in the universe is that none of it has tried to contact us.*
CALVIN AND HOBBES by BILL WATTERSON

A microchip consists of a combination of components and wires, through which signals can be sent or received. These wires create a linked network that directs electric currents to make a function happen.

Your body is like that microchip. It has a network of channels running within it. Energy passes through these channels as we tap into that source for any activity – be it playing, studying or eating.

If there is an imbalance in the level of energy within the body, a vicious cycle of stress, negativity and manifestation of disease can begin. Low energy (which can feel like lethargy or lack of motivation) or high disruptive energy can cause a circuit breakdown.

Because it's a cycle, it can also spin the other way. That's why stress in the human body is a common cause of other problems associated with imbalances in energy. Only when there is a balanced flow of energy through the body can the resultant output become positive and balanced.

> BALANCED ENERGY = POSITIVE OUTPUT
>
> UNBALANCED ENERGY = DISRUPTIVE OUTPUT

How do we turn this low disruptive energy into positive energy? Can this even be done?
It can. But what we need is a circuit breaker.

When there is excessive negative energy and the 'voltage' is uncontrolled, there is the possibility of a breakdown, and a circuit breaker gives the circuit rest instead of allowing a burnout to occur.

The practice of yoga is the circuit breaker that gives the mind and body rest, reducing stress.

Energy within the body moves through networks called nadis, or energy channels that carry the prana. The nadis circulate energies in the body. There are more than 74,000 nadis in the human body.

> Always wear bright and happy colours on a day when you're feeling low or stressed. The energy that a vibrant colour brings is unparalleled. Be your own source of light.

ENERGY = PRANA = LIFE FORCE

There are five types of energies. These energies are called vayus.

1. Pranavayu – energies that circulate upwards
2. Apanavayu – energies that circulate downwards
3. Samanavayu – energies around the level of the navel, working on digestion and assimilation
4. Udanavayu – energies around the throat and head, working on the mental faculties
5. Vyanavayu – energies that work on the body's circulation

The central nadi through which all the vayus find their root is the sushumna nadi, the spine. Each vayu has its own function.

The root of the spine can also uncoil an energy which is able to move up to the head. This doesn't happen for just anyone.

It was said that, during meditation, the Buddha's flow of energy had been directed through the sushumna

SPINE = SUSHUMNA = CENTRAL NADI

and had reached its peak, that is, the top of his head. As a result of this positive balanced energy reaching its zenith, he attained enlightenment or samadhi. Samadhi is nothing but a state of complete oneness.

For energies to ascend in this way, the first step is to gain enough strength to keep the back erect for a long period of time. No wonder we are always asked to sit straight by our teachers and parents! The stronger and more supple the spine is, the easier it is for energy to flow.

The second step in the process can occur only if we understand a secret of yogic science – the spine has many energy centres which need to be awakened so that energy can start flowing upwards. Upward flow of vital life force (prana) fuels the energy system of the body and keeps us fresh, sharp and dynamic.

NADIS = ENERGY CHANNELS = PRANA CARRIERS

There are seven primary energy centres or chakras along the spine.

1. Sahasrara chakra – on the top of the head
2. Agya chakra – between the eyebrows
3. Vishuddhi chakra – in the throat region
4. Anahata chakra – at the heart centre
5. Manipura chakra – at the navel
6. Swadhistana chakra – four inches above the mooladhara
7. Mooladhara chakra – at the base of the spine

These are secret doorways and we need to learn the passwords that will allow us through so that energy may climb higher and higher.

As energy ascends the spine, it stops and knocks at each chakra to inquire if the energy centre needs any vital life force and if it will allow the energy to pass through to the higher one. Each chakra is connected to an emotion or quality. The chakra emotion chart on page 29 shows the chakra that is active when we are feeling a certain way. For example, when we are happy the heart chakra or anahata chakra flows with energy. When we feel unsafe, insecure or tired our root chakra or the mooladhara chakra is depleted of energy. Each chakra enhances balanced emotions when energy flow is high in the body and unbalanced emotions when energy is low in the body.

How do we awaken these chakras?

Energy follows attention. When we direct our awareness to a particular chakra, energy follows and opens out the blocked chakras one by one. With free-flowing energy moving through these channels once again, mindful awareness sets the foundation for the energy to travel upwards from the base chakras up to the crown.

When the Buddha elevated his prana to the topmost energy centre, the sahasrara chakra, he found the inner peace he was looking for. The burning questions in his heart were answered. In both Buddhist and Vedic literature, the sahasrara chakra is symbolized by an epitome of beauty, a thousand-petalled lotus on top of the yogi's head or an image that looks like a halo.

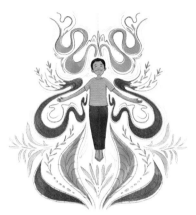

Elevated mood with flowing nadis

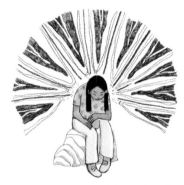

Low energy with blocked nadis

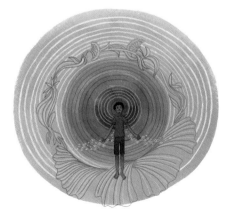

Radiating life force fuelling the chakras

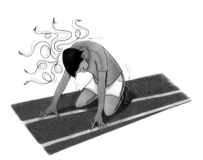

Stagnant life force shrinking the chakras

CHAKRA = ENERGY CENTRE

HAVE A FRU-GURT SUNDAE

INGREDIENTS

- Greek yogurt (or homemade yogurt)
- favourite cereal – fruit loops/corn flakes/muesli
- favourite fresh fruit – strawberries/bananas
- some jam/marmalade/jelly

HOW TO MAKE IT

Load a layer of your favourite cereal in a tall glass. Whip the yogurt and toss it in after the cereal. Follow it up with another layer of cereal, fruits and some jelly, jam or marmalade. Voila! Fru-gurt sundae for the perfect weekend breakfast is ready!

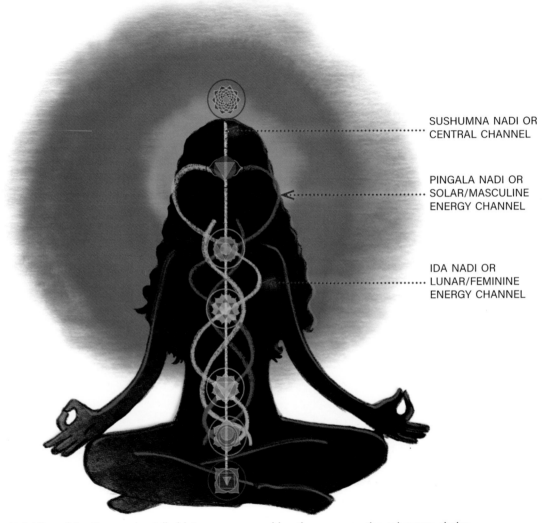

SUSHUMNA NADI OR
CENTRAL CHANNEL

PINGALA NADI OR
SOLAR/MASCULINE
ENERGY CHANNEL

IDA NADI OR
LUNAR/FEMININE
ENERGY CHANNEL

Unfolding of the thousand-petalled lotus: energy reaching the crown or the sahasrara chakra

Sahasrara chakra (crown) CONSCIOUSNESS
BALANCED: awareness, deep connection with ourselves, harmony, clarity, flow
UNBALANCED: mental fogginess, confusion, insomnia, apathy, alienation

Agya chakra (brow) LIGHT
BALANCED: focus, strong visualization, intuition, imagination
UNBALANCED: disorientation, immobility, anxiety, fatigue

Vishuddhi chakra (throat) SPACE
BALANCED: communication, self-expression, deep cleansing, detoxification, a sense of freedom
UNBALANCED: sadness, hurt, inauthenticity, invisibility, nervousness, social anxiety

Anahata chakra (heart) AIR
BALANCED: compassion, empathy, gratitude, love
UNBALANCED: loneliness, grief, sadness, jealousy, anger, pain

Manipura chakra (solar plexus) FIRE
BALANCED: control, courage, positivity, self-assurance
UNBALANCED: powerlessness, lethargy, tension, inhibition, restlessness

Swadhistana chakra (sacral centre) WATER
BALANCED: joyousness, approachability, passion, spontaneity
UNBALANCED: guilt, shame, frustration, hesitancy, self-criticism

Mooladhara chakra (root chakra) EARTH
BALANCED: security, groundedness, abundance, safety, independence
UNBALANCED: insecurity, alienation, fear, emptiness, isolation, irritation

When we are very happy, the heart chakra or the anahata chakra flows with energy.

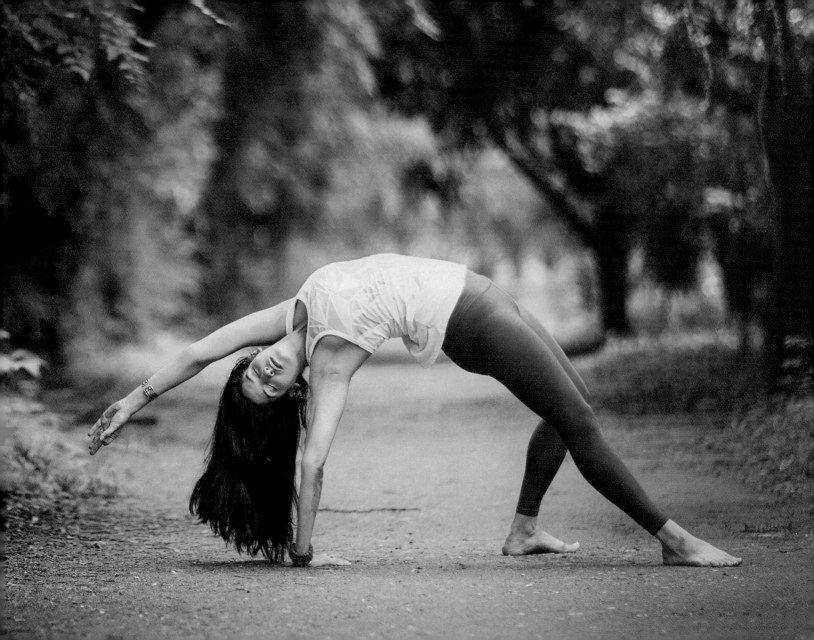

4

Mental Machinery

We are going to the moon – that is not very far. Man has so much farther to go within himself.

ANAÏS NIN
author

Think of a thread twisting. The more you twist it, the more tightly wound up it gets. There comes a point when the thread breaks.

We are like that wound-up thread when we are stressed. Every time we get anxious and irritable, we wind ourselves up and there comes a point when we just SNAP!

This usually happens when we focus too much attention on any one subject in our lives, be it study, friends or a particular goal. It is important to have these things in our lives, but if we allow any of these situations to 'stress us out' we can undermine or become blind to positives in other areas.

Ultimately, it is within our power to give our best and then take things as they come. We must remind ourselves of this daily.

Focus means the 'centre of attention'. It is good to have focus but our focus shifts as we grow and expand our horizons. At each step in life we must re-evaluate where we are and where we want to be.

Concentration is the act of being able to give your full attention to whatever is happening in the present moment. Many sages have said that equal and opposing values are complementary. This means that we will be able to concentrate fully and effectively only if we know how to *de*-concentrate fully and effectively.

This is another one of life's ancient secrets. We only know the value of light when we have experienced darkness. We only recognize the value of being happy because, at some point, we have felt sad.

The purpose of yoga, tai chi, meditation or something similar is to make us happy from the inside out. Internal happiness is ours to keep. When we are content and happy from inside, focus, concentration and awareness come to us without much effort.

Now, as we already know, the human brain is the most complex machine ever created. Memory is only one of the numerous functions of the brain.

There is a lot of ongoing research on the recall of an individual, impressions on the mind and where memory is stored so that it can be accessed whenever necessary.

From a yogi's point of view, our mind can be divided into three parts – the conscious, the subconscious and the superconscious.

The conscious mind accounts for only about 10 per cent of the total. We have access to it when we are awake and moving around. It has easily accessible memory, learning capacity and our intellect. We use this conscious mind to discriminate between the good and the bad and to recall important information for the purpose of our work. When this conscious mind is given a high workload, it becomes low in energy and undergoes stress. It is bombarded with thoughts regarding things that have happened, things that have made us unhappy or the pressure of work to be completed in the future! It goes into a frenzy darting between the past and the present. To bring the mind in the present moment and 'just be' is called *meditation*.

STRESS

How can you remain calm and poised in a stressful situation?

Stress induces a 'flight or fight' response in the brain and the body acts out of fear. To be able to reverse this process, you need to reset the body into calm mode by activating the release of 'happy hormones' or endorphins in the body.

- Simply shift your attention to any thought that makes you happy and take long, deep breaths or do an activity that makes you smile.
- Increase the 'happy hormones' in the body through meditation.
- Endorphins are also released when you eat chocolate.

Your teacher gives you a deadline and you are under pressure.

Use a technique like nadi shodhana or bhramari pranayama (see next page) to increase your energy. Yoga eliminates all the confusing chatter in the mind, giving you the confidence to do things to the best of your ability.

Up to 90 per cent of our mind may be dormant during the waking state. Deep thoughts, impressions and understandings are waiting for us to access them.

Geniuses provide a glimpse into such powers. Intuitively and mysteriously, such people – some of them very young indeed – have access to parts of their minds that enable them to excel far beyond the expectations of others.

The breath unites the body and mind and creates a calming, centred focus from within. The breath is like a string and the mind, a kite. If you can control your breath, you can control the mind.

When the mind is truly balanced, it is easier for us to concentrate for longer periods of time. No amount of pushing can create focus and balance within us, yet yoga creates this energy automatically. There is no effort needed.

Samatvam yoga ucchyate, Patanjali wrote thousands of years ago. In other words, yoga or unity with yourself is what brings steadiness in the being. Those who practise yoga will be able to remain steady even when life is turbulent.

The mind can only be steadied when we become aware that we want to learn more and find a purpose larger than ourselves. To allow this desire to germinate, we must take each day as it comes.

Almost like the internet, which needs a connection or Wi-Fi to access it, meditation provides a connection or channel that helps us tap into the intuitive capabilities that are a part of our very nature.

PREPARING OUR BODIES
TO ALLOW INCREASE IN PRANA
Morning routine
We must train our minds, bit by bit, and invite clarity. Balancing energy helps us to find purpose. With an increase in prana, we can devote our energy to creating something wonderful on the canvas of life.

We need a strong foundation to lay the building blocks of habit. The strength of the foundation

MOTHER NATURE

I have bad stomach cramps when I have my period.

- Walk about 10,000 steps every day (except during your period).
- Magnesium-rich foods, such as green, leafy veggies, beetroots and their leaves and okra, are anti-inflammatory, reduce bloating and give you strength. Hot chocolate (with almond or cashew milk), almonds, chia seeds, makhana or lotus seeds, coconut milk/water are some other options. Celery, ginger and lemon juice too help reduce pain and bloating.
- A hot water pack on the painful areas, wrapped in a towel, and soaking your feet in epsom salt reduces tenderness and gives relief.
- If necessary, take vitamin, potassium or magnesium supplements under medical supervision.
- Some asanas that are helpful during periods are butterfly pose (Chapter 6), cat pose (Chapter 6) and, of course, yoga nidra (Chapter 5).

determines how much time it takes for us to crumble. So let's start from the morning.

1. What is the first thing you do in the morning? The most natural tendency is to go and wash one's face. The ancient sages knew that there was a certain heat (or pitta) and toxins that build up in the body overnight. Washing your face disperses the heat, and freshens the mind.

2. Rinsing the mouth releases trapped heat, soothes and cools the system. It is better to give your body 10–15 minutes before you start any intensive physical activity.

3. Don't forget that tongue fuzz. Cleansing that white layer on top of the tongue cleanses the

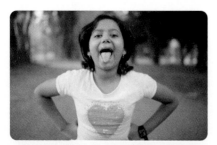
Tongue stretching

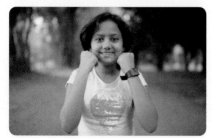
Teeth tapping

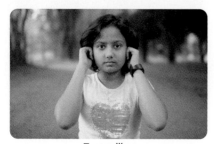
Ear pulling

ama or toxins that were generated in the body and reflected on the tongue. Scraping off the fuzz also activates one's gastric fires and gives one a refined palate as the taste buds are made more sensitive.

4. Tapping the teeth stimulates the energy channels in the mouth and strengthens the gums and enamel. Some of us chew on neem sticks which make the teeth strong and cavity-free.

5. The pressure points in the ears are connected to energy channels all over the body. Massaging the ears releases blockages and removes lethargy.

6. Bathe the right way. Bathing with cool water in the morning removes heat from the body and activates dormant energy. A bath with warm water in the evening helps with healing and relaxes the muscles.

STRENGTHENING THE SHIELD
Hakini mudra
Bring all ten fingertips together. The left and right hand mirror each other.

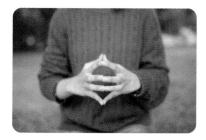

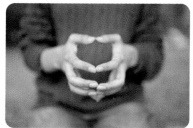

Hakini mudra

BENEFITS: Hakini mudra is said to energize your third-eye or brow centre (ajna chakra). It flushes the brain with oxygen-rich blood and improves focus and concentration. Hakini mudra also brings clarity to the mind. It is easy to do and can be done at any time, especially when you need a little inspiration.

Bhastrika

Sit in vajrasana (knees bent with the hips on the heels). Keeping the fists in front of the shoulders and elbows close to the ribcage, breathe in with strength as the palms open out above the head. Breathing out, imagine you are grabbing the stars in the sky and bring the fist back to the shoulders. Repeat another fourteen times. You can do three sets to begin with. BENEFITS: Bhastrika increases one's metabolic activity, increases lung capacity and flushes the body with positive energy that keeps you active all day long. Vajrasana after meals helps to digest food and allows for the effective absorption of nutrients in the body.

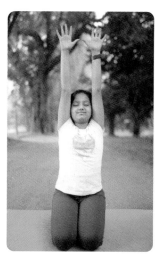

Bhastrika

Suryanamaskar

Just like the strength of the sun, suryanamaskar ignites the fire within your system.

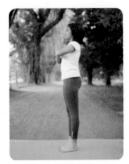

ASANA 1: Namaskar mudra or
standing salutations
MANTRA: Om mitraaya namaha

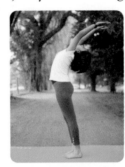

ASANA 2: Ardhachandrasana
or half moon pose
MANTRA: Om ravaye namaha

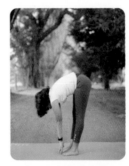

ASANA 3: Uttanasana or
Hastapadasana or forward fold
MANTRA: Om suryaya namaha

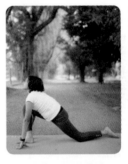

ASANA 4: Ashwasanchalasana or
horse pose
MANTRA: Om bhaanave namaha

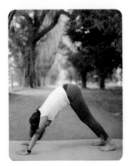

ASANA 5: Adhomukhsvanasana
or downward-facing dog pose
MANTRA: Om khagaya namaha

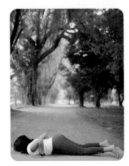

ASANA 6: Astanga namaskar
asana or 'Asta' or 8 points of
contact between body and mat
MANTRA: Om pushne namaha

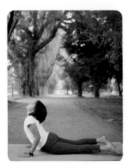

ASANA 7: Bhujangasana or
king cobra pose
MANTRA: Om hiranya namaha

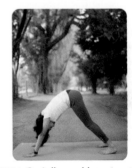

ASANA 8: Adhomukhasvanasana
or downward-facing dog pose
MANTRA: Om mareechaye namaha

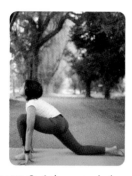

ASANA 9: Ashwasanchalasana
or horse pose
MANTRA: Om aadityaaya namaha

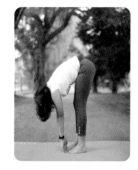

ASANA 10: Uttanasana or
standing forward bend
MANTRA: Om savitre namaha

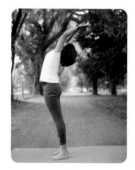

ASANA 11: Ardhachandrasana
or standing half moon pose
MANTRA: Om arkaaya namaha

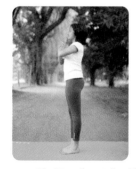

ASANA 12: Standing tall with
namaskar mudra
MANTRA: Om bhaskaraya namaha

BENEFITS: Suryanamaskar is a full-body yoga practice. It is a vinyasana, which also means 'in flow.' It is a series of twelve asanas which move every major muscle in the body.

- Brings radiance, energy and vitality in the body, much like the qualities of the sun
- Improves digestion, increases blood circulation to all the vital organs and flushes the body, brain and heart with oxygen
- Gives a glow to the skin
- Strengthens and tones the muscles in the body. You can modify the intensity and the pace of the suryanamaskar to build more muscle and enhance flexibility.
- Aids deep sleep
- Regularizes the menstrual cycle
- Reduces bloating and water retention
- Aligns the seven primary chakras in the body, especially working on the spine. If done slowly and in the correct way, suryanamaskar helps in reducing back pain.
- Builds resilience and willpower. Whenever we face an obstacle or our natural abilities meet a road block, our willpower tides us over.

Merudanda mudra

Then do merudanda mudra.

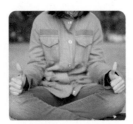

Front view

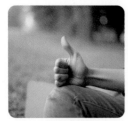 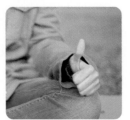

Right hand Left hand

Merudanda mudra

BENEFITS: Merudanda mudra strengthens the spine. Fill your day with things that make you happy and intersperse them with time to rest, eat and read things that nourish the self. We learn more when our minds are open to receiving from everyone and everything around us, while absorbing and extracting through trial and error what works for us and what doesn't.

Apana mudra

Touch the tips of the middle and ring fingers to the thumb. Extend the other two fingers so that they are parallel to each other. Practise this mudra for 5–10 minutes every day.

BENEFITS: Apana mudra or the mudra of digestion regulates elimination. It benefits especially those with problems of constipation and piles.

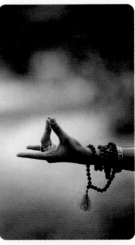

Apana mudra

There isn't any one formula, but the pieces of the puzzle are all there. It depends on you whether you want to place the pieces from out to in or the other way round. The equation you create is your own and the solution is unique too.

Once you have the solution, keep applying it every day, religiously. Finding your own answers is what makes life so interesting!

Honour everything you do. That in itself will open the doors to a smiling, healthier YOU.

DOs

1. Focus your attention inwards. Sit with your eyes closed for five minutes every day. Forget the world around you and start noticing what is happening within your mind and body.
2. Love yourself BIG time! Take care of yourself. Do things to make yourself happy.
3. Draw ALL that happy energy to you. Smile at your parents. Compliment your friends on getting that good grade.
4. Practise the act of kindness and care, every day, ALL day.

ACTIVITY

1. Close your eyes for ten minutes and listen to the many sounds around you. Note the differences in sound and see how they make you feel.
2. Play your favourite song and dance in your room like no one is watching.
3. Make all the shapes you can with sand or play dough.

Eating through the day

Why do people say we should eat a good breakfast?

The body has been asleep the last 6–8 hours and is desperately craving food that it can convert into energy. If we do not eat enough or the right food, the body will not have enough energy to play or work and muscle formation will not be complete.

Snack during study breaks.

WORK + MEDITATE + MUNCH + PLAY = MAKES TODAY A PERFECT DAY!

We know how important our favourite junk foods can be in keeping our cravings at bay. To balance them, eat something healthy at the same time – ideally home-cooked food. Feed the mind as much as the body!

Healthy eating makes for good energy that increases your attention span and memory. While studying, reach for the tuck box hidden under your bed or in your cupboard. Whether it's a few pieces of dark chocolate or cashew nuts with chaat masala, these goodies are a must! Food for the brain translates into food for thought.

Types of food

One of the sources of energy for the body is food (apart from sleep, breath and consciousness).

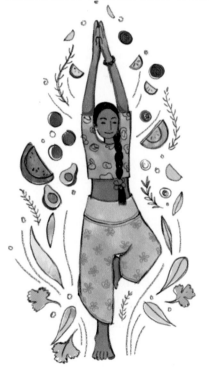

Sattvic

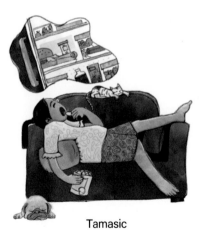

Tamasic

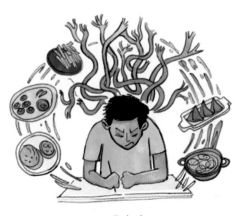

Rajasic

The energy that we get from food can be of three types depending on what we eat.

1. *Sattvic* food is high in energy and keeps the body light and the mind aware, for example, fresh fruits and vegetables.
2. *Tamasic* food makes us feel lethargic and low in energy, for example, rotten or stale food, or food with preservatives.
3. *Rajasic* food is heavy and oily. It creates a lot of activity in the mind. According to Ayurveda, excess salt or sugar can cause hyperactivity. Junk food and oily, greasy meals have the same effect.

Ancient energy-boosting herbs

- Make tea with ginger.
- Add lemongrass, licorice root, macaroot, beetroot to the ginger tea. These serve as antioxidants and immunity boosters.
- Ginseng is mostly used in its root form. It is used to convert fat into energy, to rejuvenate the mind.
- Triphala is a mix of three herbs: amalaki, haritaki and bibhitaki.

TOSSED QUINOA MADNESS

INGREDIENTS
- quinoa
- water – 2 cups
- olive oil
- onions – 2 tbsp, chopped
- garlic – 1 clove
- beans, carrots, bell peppers, mushrooms, olives, etc. – half a cup, chopped
- salt
- lime juice

HOW TO MAKE IT

Add 1 cup of raw quinoa to 2 cups of water for around 15 to 20 minutes and bring to a boil to make the quinoa dry but fluffy. Fluff out with a fork. In another pan, let onions sweat by drizzling a little salt on them for 10 minutes. Add the vegetables, garlic, etc., and sauté till the veggies are half cooked. Add the quinoa and toss it well. Add a little lime juice and salt according to taste. Garnish with a few mint leaves before serving.

TIP: Make your quinoa as colourful as possible!

SWEET POTATO CHIPS

INGREDIENTS

- sweet potatoes, washed and peeled – 2–3
- extra virgin olive oil – 2 tbsp
- thyme – a sprig
- oregano – a sprinkle
- salt – ¾ tsp
- pepper – a pinch

HOW TO MAKE IT

Preheat the oven to 250 degrees F (21 °C). Cut the sweet potatoes into thin slices. Spread them on a baking tray. Drizzle olive oil on them and place a few thyme leaves. Add salt, pepper and oregano to taste. Bake till golden brown.

- Raisins/kishmish are said to increase the coordination between the mind and the heart.
- Dates are believed to pacify the imbalance of energy in the body.

Fun with food

Here are some goodies to load yourself up with (best eaten fresh).

- Try fresh buttermilk (put a pinch of turmeric), juice or yogurt smoothies (some cinnamon thrown in).
- Oats, millets or dalia (there are different types available), quinoa, vermicelli, idli can be eaten with chopped vegetables or yogurt with fresh fruits.
- A sandwich with cucumbers, tomatoes and lettuce with cheese drizzled on top never hurt anyone!
- Meals should have vegetables of all colours supplemented with pulses and grains. So, if you're making your own whole wheat pasta, don't forget to chop those lovely red, yellow and green bell peppers and all your favourite toppings!

- Some delicious energy-boosting foods are sweet potatoes, apples, quinoa, millets, yogurt and lentils. Try sweet potato chips with home-made tomato ketchup (see Chapter 7) with your movie this weekend.

ACTIVITY: Can you identify what you eat during the day as per these three categories?

MEAL	BREAKFAST	LUNCH	DINNER
What did I eat?			
How much?			
What kind of energy did it have?			

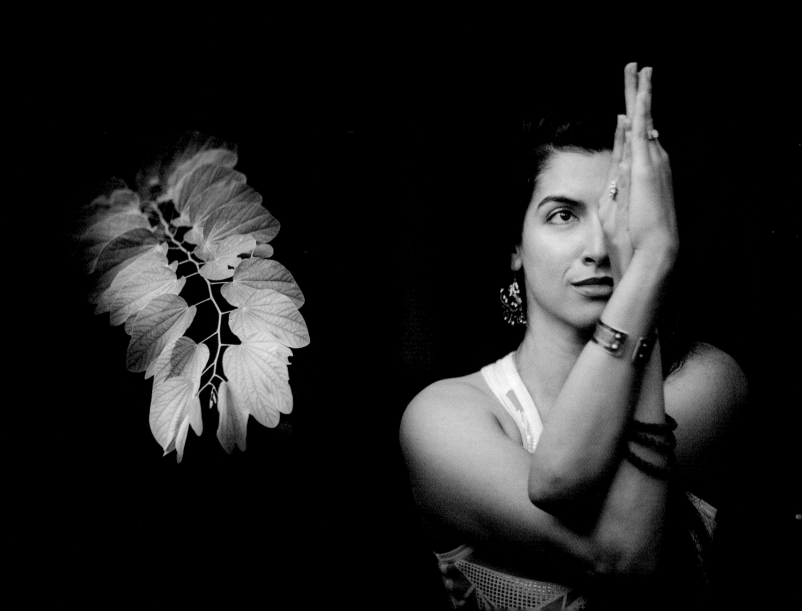

5

Daily Practices to Boost Energy

We didn't realize we were making memories,
we just knew we were having fun.
THE HOUSE AT POOH CORNER by A.A. MILNE

There is an ancient saying: One cannot pour from an empty cup. You must take care of yourself first, fill your mind and body with energy and nurture it with love. Direct kindness towards yourself before you can extend the same care to others. Life becomes more complete as you fill your cups with ojas.

Ojas is the deep reserve of vital life force that exists around you but is invisible to the naked eye. To understand how much of it you already possess, you need to observe your energy levels throughout the day. Ask yourself:

How am I feeling?

Do I feel energetic?

Do I smile often?

If you are tired, angry, restless, unhappy, cranky or miserable about anything in particular, you need to ask yourself, 'What do I need? How can I regenerate myself?' When you feel tired or sad, the level of ojas in the body is usually low. When you feel happy, light and energetic, ojas is being regenerated and levels are going up! The rays of the sun, the food you eat and the physical activity you do give you the energy to increase your connection with the nurturing and healing powers of nature.

This regeneration or boost needs to be taken in regular doses so that you keep your mind stress-free and cool while facilitating the strengthening of your body. As you begin to feel growth and radiance from within, it becomes easier to find energy to do more for yourself.

In the beginning, you may need a little more encouragement and motivation but soon you will realize that you simply need regulated breathing practices and movements to help support the goals, ambitions and dreams you are working towards. These tools will keep you going – even when the going gets tough.

ACTIVITY: Try this vision board activity. Start writing a journal. Jot down all your goals and everything you are grateful for. Add pictures, text, colours or whatever you need to give your vision more detail. Review your goals every week.

In the *Yoga Sutras of Patanjali*, one of the sutras is *Ek tattva abhyasa*. This means that a disciplined lifestyle with single-minded focus (100 per cent effort directed towards one goal) enables the mind to become whole. With an undivided mind, you can reach your destination and attain strength and clarity. Indecision, confusion and worry dissipate. Being disciplined doesn't mean not having fun. Discipline means a balanced life – enjoy what you do and take time to learn different things. For example, if you are learning how to use your left hand to brush your teeth, it will seem awkward for a few days, but if you practise consistently and regularly without a break, it becomes natural.

Whether you practise yoga, train for a sport, sing or dance, the key is focus. Energy by itself is not enough. Energy needs to be channelled in order to perfect whatever you do. Remember, energy follows attention. Think of your 'energy' as a cute puppy and 'attention' as the owner. If you focus your attention on positive goals – getting better at coding or art or maybe a sport that you want to ace – energy will

FRIENDSHIP

I feel guilty about doing well in class because my friend barely scrapes through.

- Empaths feel another person's pain or disappointment much more than other people do. Recognize that you are a sensitive person.
- Acknowledge the hard work that you have put into getting the scores you get.
- Offer to be there for your friend if they ever need to talk, discuss or even work on something together.
- You can teach them the bhramari pranayama (see later in this chapter) for a powerful memory and better concentration!

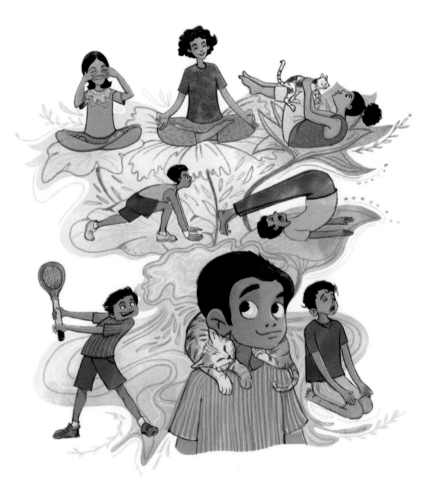

When the mind runs helter-skelter

- Research shows that an individual actively thinks about 6000 thoughts a day.
- Meditation boosts brain power. It not only improves efficiency in your work, it increases attention span and memory, relaxes you and improves the structure and functioning of the brain.
- Listening to music has been shown to positively impact language development, creativity, motor coordination, self-confidence, social and team skills, discipline, relaxation – more so in children and young people.

follow. You can transform into something better than you are. You will think empowering thoughts. You will allow yourself to feel grateful for all that you have and evolve into someone who has their feet firmly planted on the ground while your vision soars into the sky.

Now, how can you apply this energy? Vasco da Gama found a sea route to India in 1498 after sailing for one whole year. Usain Bolt succeeded in becoming the fastest man on earth after many health challenges. It was their purpose, their calling. It is important to create goals to channel your energy.

BRAIN and MIND

The brain is a part of the physical body. The mind is defined as the 'element of a person that enables them to think and feel'. The mind is much larger than the body and brain.

The mind is like a monkey that wants to run around. To contain it, you need to train it through repeated action. You need structure and consistency to keep the mind laser-focused.

The brain, however, needs to be fed with new things daily to keep it active and alert. Studies prove that if we are constantly learning new things throughout our lives, the ageing of the brain is slower. New brain connections or neural pathways are created every time you learn a new instrument, a new sport or solve a new math problem!

Do you see how the mind and brain are different? One needs to be controlled and disciplined and the other needs to be challenged every day.

The *conscious mind* constitutes only around 10 per cent of what your brain knows while you are fully awake. This knowledge could be in the form of memories, information received through observation of the environment, learnt patterns, analytical skills and interactions from what you have learnt. What you know in the 'now' comes from the conscious mind.

The *subconscious mind* is where deep information is stored. You may not even remember this information but it remains stored unconsciously in the brain. This information could include past impressions, emotions, trauma or information that might resurface if

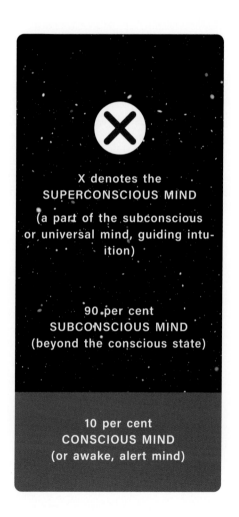

X denotes the
SUPERCONSCIOUS MIND
(a part of the subconscious
or universal mind, guiding intuition)

90 per cent
SUBCONSCIOUS MIND
(beyond the conscious state)

10 per cent
CONSCIOUS MIND
(or awake, alert mind)

something triggers a thought. For example, when you look at a blue bicycle and suddenly remember that childhood incident where you fell off on your first attempt to cycle! That information was stored in your mind but you didn't remember it till *this* moment. Fears that manifest themselves in the form of dreams also form a part of the subconscious mind.

There is an even deeper part of the subconscious mind called the *superconscious mind*. This is often referred to as the *sixth sense*. Your brain may simply know something that is beyond your observation and experience. This is something sensed, not learnt. You can tap into the powers of the superconscious mind and pull out any information you need. The superconscious mind is like the internet, from which information is downloadable – think yogis on mountains, and psychics and mentalists who read the audience's mind.

CONCENTRATION, FOCUS, MEMORY, MEDITATION

Concentration is the ability to give our 100 per cent to the priority right now. In the Mahabharata,

BRAIN

resides in the physical body, and has a definite shape, size and function which can be strengthened and enhanced through daily activity and new learnings.

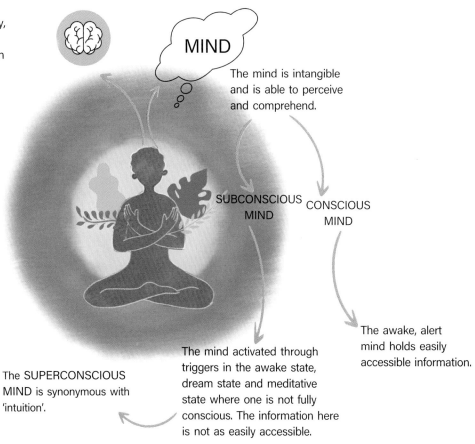

MIND

The mind is intangible and is able to perceive and comprehend.

SUBCONSCIOUS MIND

CONSCIOUS MIND

The awake, alert mind holds easily accessible information.

The mind activated through triggers in the awake state, dream state and meditative state where one is not fully conscious. The information here is not as easily accessible.

The SUPERCONSCIOUS MIND is synonymous with 'intuition'.

Brain and mind

Dronacharya, the teacher of the Kauravas and the Pandavas, asks his pupils to shoot into the eye of a bird in a tree. He asks Arjun what he sees in front of him. Unlike his peers, who say they can see the trees, leaves, sky, etc., Arjun replies he can only see the eye of the bird. That kind of determined attention takes time to build and one has to make an effort to establish such a zone.

Focus is essentially a priority or centre of interest that keeps changing according to the time and the situation. It is like a bullseye that flows and moves through the ups and downs in our lives.

When one's concentration is channelled enough to be completely in the present moment, *memory* or the power of recall is perfect.

Through *meditation* we can tap into the superconscious mind or sixth sense at will. The power of meditation can accelerate us towards all that we want in our lives and all that we want to give to our world. It is like our wishbone or our four-leaved clover.

THE PRINCIPLES OF CONCENTRATION

The mind is much larger than the body. An untamed mind can be described as wild horses all pulling in different directions – restless and overwhelmed with thoughts. One can also think of the mind like a monkey, jumping from thought to thought. Your monkey mind pulls pranks on you and often makes you do stuff that you just don't realize.

- It makes you fear or worry about things even if they never happen.
- It makes you run after unimportant things that may seem important in the moment: you get really restless to watch the next season of your favourite series releasing on Netflix just the day before your history exam. It can take you away from doing the deep work you need to do.
- It pulls you in many directions by thinking and can often confuse you – should you get that Belgian chocolate ice cream or the Nutella waffles for dessert? The quality of your decisions, big or small, is determined by the quality of your thought process.

CONCENTRATION, *noun*
the action or power of focussing all one's attention, attentiveness or centralization

FOCUS, *noun*
centre of interest or activity, the focal point, central point, hub, pivot, nucleus, emphasis or priority

MEMORY, *noun*
the power of recall or the ability to remember

MEDITATION, *noun*
a practice in which an individual uses a technique, such as mindfulness or focussing the mind on a particular object, thought or activity, to train attention and awareness, and achieve a mentally clear and emotionally calm and stable state

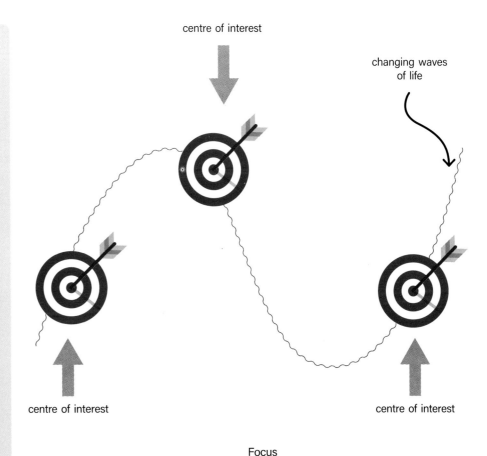

centre of interest

changing waves of life

centre of interest

centre of interest

Focus

- It makes you daydream and put off doing things until the last minute.
- The mind can distract you or be your powerhouse depending on how you use it. It can be a blunt pencil or a sharp one. If there is laser focus on your goal, one can learn to prioritize what they choose to work towards with clarity. Then even going to watch an *Avengers* movie will come second to that swimming practice you had scheduled.

How can you decode the mind? How do you become its master instead of the other way round?

A yogi or a seeker is one who is always ready to embrace knowledge and apply it – always wanting to know more. However, when you meditate, you are doing the opposite of concentration. You are learning to just be. Relax. Do nothing.

When you stop fighting and resisting your thoughts, the mind stops fighting back. When you calm down, the mind rests too. Through meditation, you can relax the mind and direct its energies as needed. When you sit still in meditation with a question, sometimes there is an automatic information download. Your mind is able to see a situation with clarity and you can process this information by tapping into a higher version of yourself which is then able to guide you.

Hence, *de*-concentration or meditation is the science of being effortlessly aware. It is the key to a whole new world.

However, before you begin to meditate effortlessly, you need to know the other side of the coin too. Only when you learn to concentrate can you experience *de*-concentration! To think out of the box, you first need to be *in* the box.

Let us learn how to concentrate to be able to work efficiently! And *de*-concentrate to be able to relax completely. You can use these tools as and when you need to.

How do we decode and de-concentrate?

The one thread that connects the mind and the body is the breath. When you learn how to control the breath, the mind and body will naturally come into sync.

DE + CONCENTRATION = MEDITATION

Have you noticed how easy it is to sync your tablet to your phone or your laptop? You just need to know how to do it, right? The correct technique.

It is the same with breath, only simpler. When you run somewhere or are afraid or worried about an outcome, your breathing becomes heavy, fast and short. Conversely, when you are happy, you are able to take long, deep and relaxed breaths. The monkey mind can be reined in with a few simple techniques. So, every time you get restless, try the following.

Anuloma viloma (nadi shodhana or alternate nostril breathing)

TECHNIQUE: Start by exhaling completely from the left nostril. Inhale from the left again to begin the sequence and exhale from the right. Inhale from the right and exhale from the left. Each round starts and ends with the left nostril.

BENEFITS: This is an ancient technique that activates the pituitary gland, balances the left and the right brain and enhances memory. Research has proven that inclusion of

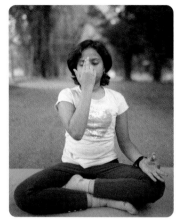
Alternate nostril breathing

alternate nostril breathing in the daily exercise regimen is very beneficial for cognitive development.

The right nostril is considered the solar nostril (regulating the level of heat in the body) and the left is the lunar nostril (regulating how the body cools down).

The body is like your home. Imagine if the air conditioning or the heater was broken; the rooms would get too hot or too cold for comfort. Similarly, when we have a cold or a blocked nose, we cannot breathe comfortably and experience a heavy head. Alternate nostril breathing gets the body's natural heat and cooling factors in balance so that the body doesn't feel that it is under attack and its temperature and immunity remain optimal. This practice also balances the flurry of activity in the mind to leave you relaxed and calm.

Bhramari pranayama

TECHNIQUE: Using the index finger to shut the inner flap of the ear, make a buzzing sound that reverberates in the head keeping your lips closed. Do this around 3–5 times to begin with, working it up to 21 times.

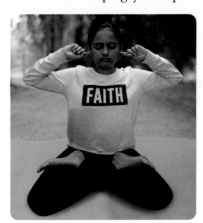

Bhramari pranayama

BENEFITS: Bhramari activates the parasympathetic nervous system, reduces excessive thoughts, increases concentration and brings you out of 'fight or flight' mode. For many of you who have sleepless nights before exams and worry that you will forget everything, bhramari is the perfect memory booster. It has a profoundly beneficial impact on mental health.

Power nap or yoga nidra

TIP: Ask a parent or a study buddy to help. It can be done alone too, but it is always better to start with someone guiding you.

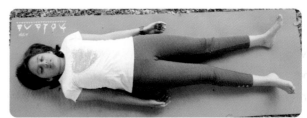

Yoga nidra or deep yogic sleep

TECHNIQUE: Start by lying down on your back in shavasana. Let your partner instruct you to guide your breath through the different parts of your body starting with the right leg, left leg, hip, back, stomach, chest, arms, neck and head. Spend a few moments on each body part with the feeling of gratefulness and calm. Keep breathing long and gently through the process. Allow the mind to relax.

BENEFITS: Yoga nidra increases anabolic processes in the body which heal and repair the system, produce greater calm and relaxation, rejuvenate the mind and allow deeper and more restful sleep.

JUST BE YOURSELF

Too much to do and too little time is the bane of every student's existence. You want to do your best and this is only possible when you are connected and calm within. Every aspect of learning comes together – whether it is focus, concentration or memory. Meditation and breathing techniques are the easiest ways of bringing out your hidden, unique and dynamic qualities.

> ACTIVITY: Take an object – a glass or a pen, anything at all. Now focus all your attention on this object. Observe all the details – the colour, shape, texture, etc. After five minutes, write down as many details as you can remember.

Meditation is a process of letting go. Of course, if this were as easy as celebrities make it out to be then wouldn't we all be doing this? Who wouldn't like to have the resilience and confidence of Virat Kohli or play badminton like P.V. Sindhu?

The truth is, it isn't very difficult and you needn't spend long hours to master meditation.

1. Begin by focussing on something external or internal. External focus could be attention to a pen or cloud, an empty wall, a blade of grass, a bird, your own hand, feet, mirror-gazing into your eyes or even someone's head. (Sounds strange, right? But this step will help you slip into the meditative state a little more easily.) Just about any object or person that you see can be a part of this external focus. Choose only one at a time. Internal focus can be on your own third eye centre, your breath, a thought or visual.

2. De-concentrate and relax. Once you've got your focus in place, start watching yourself and how you are feeling. Sometimes old thoughts pop up, sometimes random dreams about the future,

SLEEP CHALLENGES

My mind becomes even more active at night. I go to bed at 10 p.m. every day but don't fall asleep till at least two hours later. I don't wake up fresh in the morning.

- Switch off the phone half an hour before going to bed. The blue light keeps the brain awake and reduces melatonin (a hormone that induces sleep cycles and the natural rhythms of the body).
- If the mind is very active, asanas such as marjariasana and pawanmuktasana (Chapter 6) help to ease the tightness in the neck, spine and back.
- Bhramari pranayama has a calming impact on the mind. It has been shown to activate melatonin, which helps the mind to unwind and helps the body heal during deep rest.
- Massaging your temples with peppermint oil is very soothing for the nerves. You can also put a few drops of it on your pillow.
- Yoga nidra is another powerful tool that you could use.

sometimes bizarre thoughts that have no connection and there are moments when you might feel this floaty state where no thoughts buzz around your head. This is the 'nothingness space' you want to get to. Many of us experience this very differently but with some similar characteristics. Meditation can leave you sleepy, energetic, smiling or sad. The most important thing it teaches you is to face every emotion that comes into your life. As you practise meditation every day, you become strong from within. You become a gentle warrior.

KINDS OF MEDITATION

1. *Breath meditation* – a gentle focus on one's breathing patterns before moving into an effortless, relaxed state.
2. *Walking meditation* – attentive walking with one's mind completely soaked in the present moment and one's surroundings.
3. *One-pointed focus meditation* – focussing on a subject of choice and keeping our awareness there for as long as possible; initially focus on an external point and gradually, as you get better, focus on an internal, non-tangible point.
4. *Progressive muscle relaxation* – taking your awareness to each muscle one by one and relaxing that area, sitting or lying.
5. *Yoga nidra* – a meditation that works on progressive relaxation in a lying down position, as you've already read. There are many beginner, intermediary and advanced yoga nidra techniques with visualization.
6. *Mantra meditation* – brings the mind into a relaxed, stress-free state by using a mantra or sound repeatedly.
7. *Guided visualization* – guided relaxation techniques that help not only settle the numerous thoughts in the mind but also help one face internal struggles, challenges, fears, doubt, grief and other emotional upheavals by creating release.
8. *Mindfulness meditation* – accepting and being mindful of 'what is' instead of what can be.

These are some of the oldest ways to meditate. When you start practising, you might find some recurring themes in many of these meditation methods.

Even starting with ten minutes of meditation every day goes a long way and creates permanent changes in the brain's physiology and one's approach to life. Research has shown that with even as little as two weeks of regular meditation, one can start seeing changes in one's state of mind.

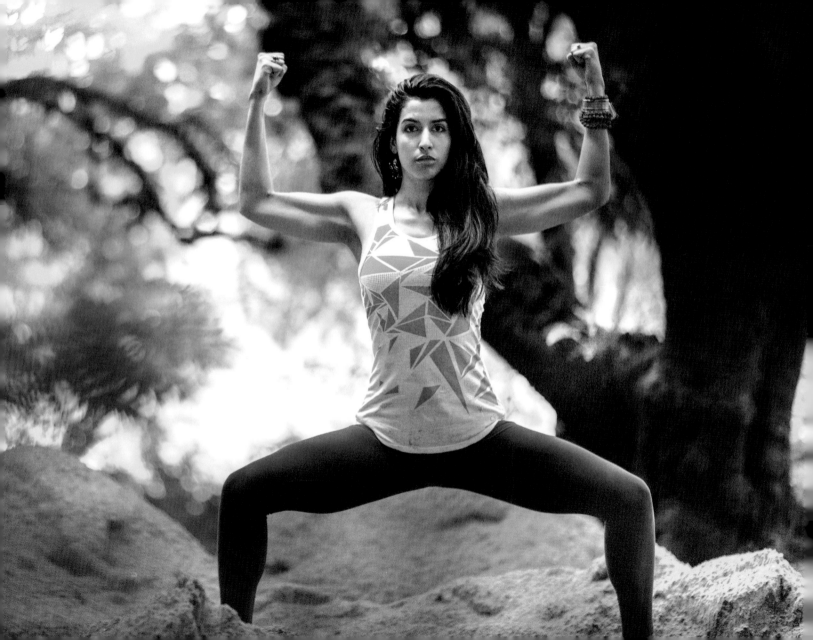

6

The Budding You

It's not where you go;
it's who you meet along the way.
THE WIZARD OF OZ by L. FRANK BAUM

Maturing is natural but growing up is optional. We learn through experience. Through trial and error, we learn to adapt and create a path for ourselves.

When young, we constantly hear people tell us to become more 'responsible' – make our bed, feed our pets and so forth. The workload expected of us becomes heavier as the years pass, particularly with the increasing demands of school life. But there is no need to be crushed by the pressure of it all.

When you have a truckload of things to do, remember:

1. There will be some things that you can do at your own pace. Remember the 'slow and steady wins the race' adage? But this doesn't mean you keep postponing!

2. Asking for help doesn't make you look weaker. In fact, you make more meaningful relationships when you reach out to people. Be ready, in turn, to extend a helping hand yourself!

3. Avoid thinking that the world is on your shoulders and take time to breathe and unwind by using breathing tools and meditating a little between tasks. Any yogi's archnemesis is stress. So, be sure to smile in the face of adversity and say, 'Not now, not ever!'

4. Growing up doesn't mean just growing in size. It means learning to make sense of the world before us. A true yogi is not one who can stand on his head but one who is kind and compassionate and strong enough to navigate through tough situations, especially if they scare us.

Setting your own priorities and making decisions, especially when others will judge you for them, are a part of growing up. As young children, you are told what you must do. The simplest way of assessing an action you might wish to take is to ask yourself these questions:

Will it really make me happy?

Will I be harming anyone or myself if I take this action?

If the answer to either of these questions is 'No' or 'I don't know', you know you need to take a step back and re-evaluate your course of action. A little more mulling over the situation before you make your decision might be a good idea.

The strength to do what is right defines the kind of 'grown up' you are. Taking responsibility for your actions does not mean that you can't be happy and responsible at the same time. A responsible person is also responsible for their own health and happiness.

Even if life is chaotic, the effort to create a haven of serenity for yourself is more important than achieving all the #lifegoals on the planet.

Find that one thing you can keep coming back to whenever life throws a curveball at you (and that doesn't mean eating chocolate or spending hours playing video games). It might be painting, playing a sport, climbing trees, gardening, cuddling your cat, talking to a friend or a therapist or standing upside down. Work with your hands and keep the energy flowing. The closer you stay to the earth and the outdoors, the more energy you absorb from nature. Take time out to do something outdoors every day.

A little child-like excitement is what keeps the fun in life (as long as you're not ignoring the work bit). And a sense of purpose in life is what makes it all worthwhile.

Fuel for the brain!

VEGAN DATE SHAKE
INGREDIENTS
- pitted dates – 5–6
- water/milk/milk substitute – a glass
- almonds – 10

HOW TO MAKE IT
Soak the almonds overnight. Peel the skin of the almonds in the morning. Toss in the peeled almonds with a glass of milk/milk substitute/ water (in case of allergies). Blend in the mixer till all granular bits have dissolved. Add pitted dates for sweetness and blitz again. Serve fresh.
TIP: Best not to strain.

Whether making new friends or learning how to skate, each step you take brings you one step closer to knowing yourself better. Ultimately, that may be what growing up is all about – understanding yourself a little better than you did before.

Growing up means being sensitive to your environment. It means making your own decisions, and that means you can do something different – you can make your life, with all its ups and downs, a thrilling roller-coaster ride.

GROW UP, GLOW UP

When the mind feels fuzzy or there is a big decision to make, these are the asanas to help you activate the parasympathetic nervous system (the cooling network) and harness the power of your brain.

The following asanas are especially effective if you're in the process of puberty. These postures support you if your voice is getting heavier, your body is changing or when you have your period or have painful periods. These asanas are safe for those with polycystic ovary syndrome too. You can do the full sequence or pick a few.

Seated body rotation

TECHNIQUE: Sit comfortably with your legs crossed and the spine straight. Keep your palms on your knees. With a long breath in, slowly lean back and, as you exhale, move the body forward bringing the

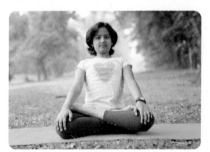
Step 1

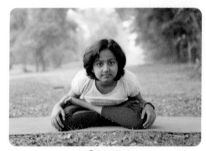
Step 2

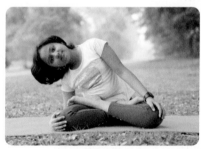
Step 3

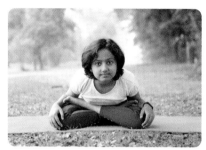

Step 4

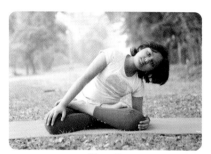

Step 5

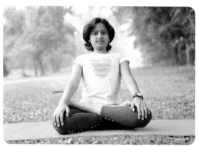

Step 6

nose as close to the floor as you can without strain. Start moving the spine in large circles, breathing in as you go back half circle and exhaling as you move the body through the other half. Do five rounds clockwise and five rounds anti-clockwise.

BENEFITS: It relaxes the muscles of the lower back and sides, reducing any pain that might be present. Focusing on the breath induces calm and relaxation of the nervous system.

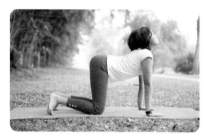

Step 1

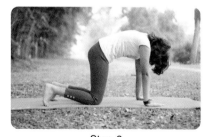

Step 2

Marjariasana

Marjariasana (cat pose)

TECHNIQUE: Get on all fours. Breathing in, move your head back, stretching the throat. Note that the stomach pushes down; the spine moves into a convex shape and looks like a bowl. Next, exhale slowly and touch your chin to your chest, raising the spine like a camel's hump. Then, straighten the spine into the neutral position. Repeat ten times.

BENEFITS: It relaxes the entire spine and the core of the nervous system, which is deeply embedded along the spine. It regulates the sympathetic and parasympathetic nervous system. Marjariasana not only makes the body flexible but also strengthens the arms and shoulders while stretching the stomach and easing any discomfort in this region. It activates the thyroid gland which helps stabilize body and weight fluctuations. This asana is very effective in relieving back pain during periods.

Kurmasana (tortoise pose)
TECHNIQUE: Sit up and stretch your legs out in a seated position. Bend your knees and bring your feet

to the floor. Widen the feet to twice the width of your shoulders. Slide your arms under the knees. Gently drop your body forward. Try and touch your nose to the ground. Stretch your arms out on either side. You are like a tortoise in its shell! Hold for ten breaths and slowly find your way back into the seated position.

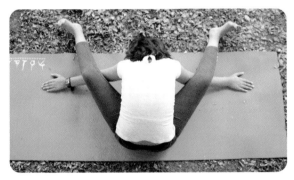

Kurmasana

BENEFITS: This asana for hip and spinal flexibility helps in neck and shoulder pain or stiffness, strengthens the arms, legs, abdomen and pelvis, helps in constipation and improves lung capacity. It's a great asana to do after your dance workout or football practice.

Baddhakonasana (butterfly pose)
TECHNIQUE: Join the soles of the feet and pull the heels close to the hips in sitting position. Keep the spine straight. Flap the knees on either side with equal force 10–20 times and then gradually bring the head towards the toes. Hold for as long as you can. Relax.

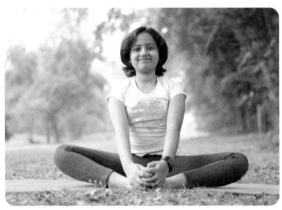

Baddhakonasana

BENEFITS: The butterfly pose brings a sense of lightness in the body. It opens out the hip flexors and creates greater mobility in the lower back and erector-spinae muscles.

Bhujangasana (cobra pose)

TECHNIQUE: Lie down on your stomach. Keep the palms on either side of the chest. Keep the heels joined together. Breathing in slowly, lift the chest off the ground till the navel. The elbows can remain bent but the heels must remain together. Exhaling, slowly bring the chest back to the ground.

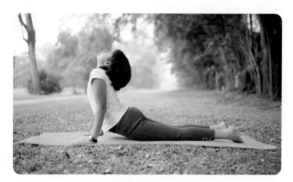

Bhujangasana

BENEFITS: Regular practice of this pose not only strengthens the upper body and back but also creates a spine as supple as the king cobra. It regulates the different glands in the body including the pituitary, which is the master gland controlling all hormones secreted into the system. Whenever you feel overwhelmed, try stretching in Bhujangasana and breathe!

Ardhashalabhasana (locust pose)

TECHNIQUE: Lie down on your stomach, hands straight by the side of the body, palms facing the ground. Breathing in, slowly raise the right leg off the ground keeping the knee straight. Exhaling gradually, bring the right leg down and relax. Repeat with the left leg. Hold each leg up for 8–10 breaths.

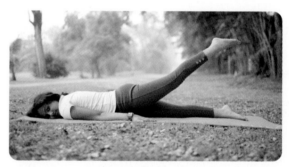

Ardhashalabhasana

BENEFITS: This asana is helpful for strengthening the back and easing sciatica pain. It works on correcting the imbalance in cervical spondylosis and removes any excess weight around the hips and thighs. Shalabhasana (with both legs) helps bring balance and strength in the lower body, just as bhujangasana does for the upper body.

Pawanmuktasana (air balancing pose)

TECHNIQUE: Lie on your back. Stretch your legs out. Keeping the neck and head pressed into the floor, raise the right knee, bend it and bring it as close to the chest as you can. Hug the right knee with both hands and slowly raise your nose towards the knee. Pull the toes of the right foot towards your body and push the thigh and knee of the left leg flat on the ground. Repeat with the other leg. Hold each side for 8–10 breaths.

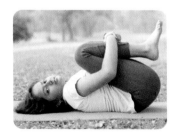 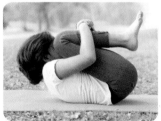

Step 1   Step 2

Pawanmuktasana

BENEFITS: This asana stretches the neck and back. The abdominal muscles are tensed and the internal organs are compressed, which increases blood circulation and stimulates the nerves, increasing the efficiency of the internal organs. The pressure on the abdomen releases any trapped gases in the large intestine. This reduces any gas or feeling of bloating in the body.

Supt Natrajasana (reclining lord of the fish pose)

TECHNIQUE: Start by lying down on your back with your legs stretched out. Keep both hands at shoulder level. Breathing in, lift the right leg and place it on the left knee. Taking the left hand, place it on the right knee. Keep the right shoulder glued to the floor. Breathing out, slowly drop the right knee towards your left side, assisted by the left hand, look towards the right hand. Feel the stretch on the hips, thighs and the spine. Repeat on the other side. Hold for 8–10 breaths.

BENEFITS: Supt Natrajasana stretches the hips and quadriceps. As you twist, there is a certain amount of pressure on the abdominal organs which increases

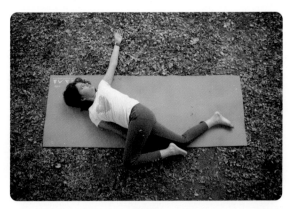

Right

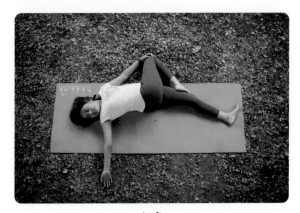

Left

Supt Natrajasana

blood circulation and improves their functioning, thereby improving digestion and immunity. This asana relaxes the body and induces calm and relaxation.

Vajrasana (thunderbolt pose)

TECHNIQUE: Sit with your hips on the heels. Make sure your toes do not overlap. Breathe for 3–4 minutes in this posture.

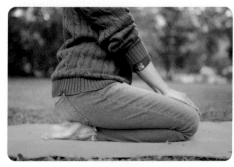

Vajrasana

BENEFITS: The practice of this asana reduces bloating in the stomach, improves digestion, increases blood circulation and strengthens pelvic floor muscles. This asana induces restful sleep before bedtime if combined with deep breathing.

FRIENDSHIP

I can't say no even to my friend when I don't want to do something.

Boundaries are important. Don't feel obliged to do anything that doesn't make you feel comfortable. Express your feelings instead of shutting down. Take time to think things over before committing and saying yes. A few things you can say to your friend (in your own words):

- Thank you for being my friend, but there are some decisions I have to make on my own.
- Thank you for respecting my decision of not moving ahead with this.
- I am not comfortable with what you're asking me to do. This doesn't change how I view our friendship. I will always be there to support your decisions and when you want to share your thoughts.
- I understand that we can have different perspectives. I respect your decision to go ahead, without judgement.

Back pain mudra

TECHNIQUE: Focus your attention on your left hand. Bring the thumb and index finger together in chinh mudra. On the right hand, bring the tip of the little finger, middle finger and thumb together. This is known as the back pain mudra.

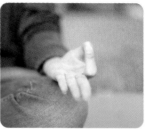

Left-hand view 1   Left-hand view 2

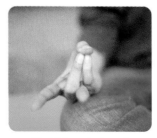
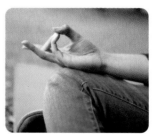

Right-hand view 1   Right-hand view 2

Back pain mudra

Have you noticed how listening to instrumental music can relax you or make you feel sleepy? Rock music and hip-hop makes you 'amp up' a little when you go for a run or exercise? Music has the power to shift your mood. When you are feeling sad, play a happy song to lift your spirits! Research talks about how learning musical skills directly impacts language development, creativity, motor coordination, self confidence, social and team skills, discipline, relaxation and more in children and young people.

BENEFITS: This mudra works on relieving discomfort anywhere along the spine, neck and shoulders. Lower back pains are common when we are growing rapidly. Use this mudra whenever you need it. You can even do it lying down in bed.

Whenever you experience periods of restlessness and fluctuation of energy, make sure you are resting enough.

According to Patanjali, the sixth pillar of yoga is dharana, that is, 'one-pointed attention'. Dharana teaches you to sit and focus. When you can contain your focus and solidify it, you can retain your awareness for long periods of time.

Just as a pupa experiences rest within its cocoon before it turns into a beautiful butterfly, you transform into a subtle, thoughtful and powerful individual each time you go through the transformative process. Whether it is reaching puberty or leaving the nest on your own, the whole world is your oyster! Every time there is a challenge in your life, you grow better, stronger and more aware.

Be it your relationships, expectations, desires or wants, you have the power to channel your thoughts to live the best life within and without. Life's challenges are what make this journey so eventful!

ACTIVITY: Taking responsibility
- Find a cause you are passionate about and throw a fundraiser.
- Learn to cook. You can start by making some of the recipes in this book.
- Manage your pocket money well – learn to spend on necessities and save. That way, any treats you receive from others will mean a lot more.
- Look after your physical and mental health by doing exercise of some kind every day, such as asanas, pranayama and meditation, as discussed in this book.

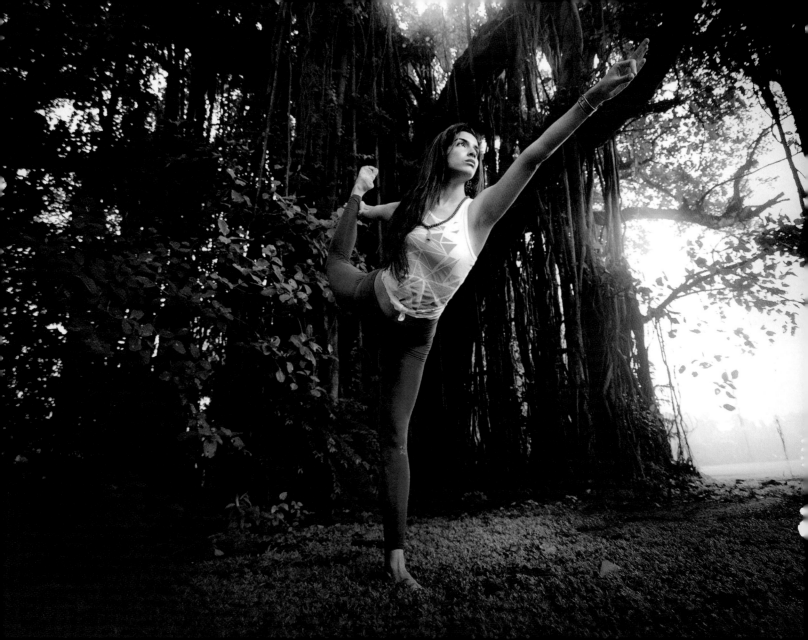

7

Believing in Balance

*Happiness is when what you think, what you say
and what you do are in harmony.*

MAHATMA GANDHI
prominent leader and freedom fighter

Some days in life seem almost magical. Other days, everything seems to go wrong.

Imagine waking up feeling great. The world looks beautiful. Birds are chirping outside your window and you've got plans. Then your mother walks in and says that you're late. Not only that, but you need to clean your room. Part of you gets annoyed, but you still go off to school expecting your favourite sandwich or pao bhaji in your tiffin box. Instead, you find a mass of soggy green with chapatis. You are probably irritated by now. Then you look for your regular seat on the bus on the way back and find that it has been taken by the new kid. Okay, that's the last straw! You lose your cool.

Most human beings have a tendency to attach their happiness to things, events or circumstances. We allow situations around us to dictate our feelings. We want or expect things to go our way – and we feel that our mood or emotional state depends on it.

We want to be happy but don't know how. We imagine that happiness is what happens to us as a simple consequence of nothing being or going wrong, and that, when things are not quite right, happiness is beyond our reach.

Too often, we defer happiness, making it dependent on something that may or may not happen. Too often, we place the responsibility for our happiness on someone else.

Most of us can see something of ourselves in these statements:

I'll be happy only if I get 10/10 in my class test.
I'm unhappy because I'm not cool enough, not popular enough.
I can't be happy if I don't win that prize.
If only I had been allowed to go to that party …
If only I was taller …
If only I could make everyone happy …
If only I was loved by …

When we attach happiness to external factors, the price we pay is a rollercoaster ride that has more downs than ups. We can never truly be happy because, even if one small thing goes wrong, our sense of inner peace is likely to evaporate with the hope or expectation we invested in it. Then, rest assured those

BODY IMAGE

I have started getting pimples on my face. I don't like looking at myself in the mirror. I feel tempted to pop them.

All of us experience hormonal changes in different ways.

- A balanced diet (no fried, oily, spicy or white sugary foods) can help the body combat hormonal changes so much better. Fried and sugary foods attack the immune system. Replace them with fresh, sattvic food whenever possible.
- Drink enough water every day.
- Keep your body alkaline by eating at least two pieces of fruit a day.
- Combine this with regular exercise – running, playing cricket or tennis with your friends, working out in the gym, dancing, doing yoga or any other kind of movement.
- Keep your face clean and dry. Use a dermatologist-recommended moisturizer and sunscreen. Popping pimples only spreads more bacteria!

volcanic eruptions of anger or landslides of frustration or disappointment will always be part of the emotional landscape.

It's clear, therefore, that we must try to find happiness within. How?

Growing up, we are sometimes told of the need to 'walk the middle path', and that 'life is a struggle'.

We must make constant efforts to bridge the gap between what we need and what we want.

How do we decide what is really important for us and what we can simply do away with?
The heart wants what the heart wants. Even if we try to push our desires away, there are times when our

heart simply cannot dismiss them. Wants and desires are natural, but it is important to understand that how you deal with them is your choice.

Yoga karamsu kaushalam. Yoga refines our sensibilities and gives us the skills to better handle situations, feelings and desires – the challenges of daily life. Greater self-awareness through yoga enables us to approach life with more clarity. Imagine the confidence that follows when you know that no one can push your buttons unless you allow them to! That is the power we can work towards – the power of complete belief.

When you sit and watch your thoughts, do you realize how many thoughts are actually chilling in your mind? Thoughts of food, your friends, your crush or maybe even that upcoming science test? The greatest challenge in life is dealing with the mind. While it is natural to want things, we may be on a never-ending rollercoaster without realizing it. If we cannot harness the mind, we condemn ourselves to constant distraction, and eternal dissatisfaction.

Taming the monkey mind is the most difficult task but, once we have found a way to become consistently better at it, the rewards are wonderful. When we learn how to observe our desires without chasing them, we begin to develop inner strength and willpower; our lives open up to happiness, calm and joy. We become the superheroes we are meant to be.

Meditation is food for the mind (read more about meditation in Chapter 5). Meditation and rest allow the mind to become sharper and more efficient. We feel clearer and more awake. Both states are natural and equally important for the brain to get a cleanse.

No matter how skilled we become in our practice of yoga, desires and distractions will always crop up. What do we do then?

Remember, thoughts are temporary, just like everything else. They come, and they go. It is best to simply observe the mind and what it is drawn to. Instead of trying to push unwanted thoughts away, allow them in. *What we resist persists.* Once allowed in, thoughts will linger for a while – but before you know it, they will be replaced by new ideas and other thoughts. Life is ever-changing.

Life is better when you have your 'business' and your 'busyness' sorted. Sometimes, we have so many things to do that it can feel as if we are struggling to keep our heads above water. Avoid making hurried decisions that you may regret later on. The keys here are patience and watchfulness. Develop a process to optimize time – and remember that starting quick is starting smart.

- Make a list of what needs to be done.
- Prioritize your list – most important, a little less important ... Take help from someone if you need to. Don't be afraid to reach out.
- Act on the first, most painful or overdue thing on the list. It just gets easier from there.

Believe, and you are halfway there. The strength, confidence and centred sense of being that you achieve on the yoga mat are the tools you need to blossom off the mat, in life. Embracing the practice of yoga, and making yoga a part of your deepest self will bring you that equanimity.

Samatvam yoga ucchyate. The ups and downs in life continue, challenges come and go, and all the things around you keep changing, but nothing should shake your foundations.

The next time someone gives you a tough time, will you be able to smile and remain unshaken? That is the *you* that you might become, the you that believes in being more than you ever were. How do we attain this priceless SKILL?

S = Sensible, Sensitive
K = Kind
I = Intuitive
L = Learn constantly
L = Listen and observe

Sensible, sensitive

Looking at things from an external perspective and applying judgement in context is an important skill. To be sensitive and empathize, and yet be able to hold one's own ground without unnecessary conflict is a quality worth cultivating.

Make it at home!

TOMATO KETCHUP

INGREDIENTS
- fresh tomatoes – 2 kg
- onion, grated – 1 medium-sized
- brown sugar – 2 tbsp
- extra virgin olive oil – 2 tbsp
- garlic, grated – 2 cloves
- ginger – 1" piece
- basil – a few sprigs
- bay leaf – 1

HOW TO MAKE IT

Blitz the tomatoes in a blender. Lightly heat the olive oil in a pan. Add the onion and cook till it is slightly caramelized. Add the garlic and ginger and let it simmer on medium heat. Stir continuously. Add the tomato blend, brown sugar and salt to taste. Add all the herbs/leaves and let it simmer for a while. It will take about 20 minutes to become a rich, thick, flavourful consistency. Then, simply let it cool.

Kind

Being able to reach out to those who need help and to inspire others to do the same, often as a team, is a skill that brings people together. Treat everyone with kindness and you shall always get it in return.

Intuition

Developing and honing intuition is also a result of skill and grace. Often when we are at a crossroads, having a balanced and peaceful mind activates our 'gut' instinct and leads us in the right direction.

Learn constantly

Keep an open heart and mind. Know that every day, every person and every situation teaches us something. So even if we are in a tough spot, the wise thing would be to make the most of the situation. Upgrade your understanding of the world and of yourself. Know that the tough times will change too.

Listen and observe

Each person has qualities of their own. Identify these qualities within those around you and admire them for it. The more we observe, the less we are shaken internally. We can harness true invincibility if we learn to listen and see situations without getting entangled in the moment. There is a solution to every problem, if we look at it from the outside. When we find emotional balance, we can find harmony within – and then the storm can only bend us, never break us.

The complex machine

The human brain is the most complex machine in the world. Even science is limited in its understanding of how our brain works. Each of us has a left brain and a right brain. The left side of the brain corresponds to the creative aspects of our nature and the right side governs the logical faculties. Some of us feel that at a given time we have greater creative capabilities or that we're more logical in nature. If we feel more adept at solving problems on some days and quickly send in our maths papers, or can argue efficiently with examples in our conversations, it might be that the right brain is in overdrive. On days when we are feeling inspired, needing to experiment with new ideas, the left brain may be more active. It is however possible to bring both the logical and creative sides at par, enhancing both faculties, but not without practice.

ACTIVITY: Get out of your comfort zone and say hi to someone outside your circle of friends. Make a new friend!

How do we bridge this gap between the logical and creative?

The right side of the body activates the left brain and the left side of the body activates the right brain. It's like a criss-cross. When the left and right brain are in sync with each other, we are better able to cope with challenges in our life and it is easier for us to feel at peace with ourselves.

BODY IMAGE

I am overweight and I feel self-conscious. I hear the kids sniggering at me. I don't feel like eating in front of people. All of us experience hormonal changes in different ways.

Many of us feel insecure of our ever-changing bodies. Know that you are not alone.

- Our body stores fat whenever it feels that there is a drought or shortage of food. However, if we withhold food from the body, we feel tired, weak or experience brain fog. A balanced diet makes it easier for us to maintain a healthy weight for our height and body type. It simply isn't true that all foods make us fat. Choose good food and keep your body fit.
- There may be people in our lives who make us feel uncomfortable or laugh at our choices. It is easiest to simply ignore these people. We can't run away from difficult situations; however, we can learn to stand our ground. Make informed decisions and keep your sattvic energy high.

Here are a few practices that ancient yogis performed to bring more balance in their lives and to activate intuitive powers.

Anuloma viloma

Alternate nostril breathing or nadi shodhana, as explained in Chapter 5, is one such practice.

Vrikshasana (tree pose)

TECHNIQUE: Stand tall with your feet shoulder width apart. Place your left foot on the right inner thigh/knee or calf (at a level on the right leg that is easy to balance). Focus on a point in front of you. Keep breathing easily. Do not hold your breath at any point.

ANXIETY

I find it very difficult to focus before exams. I waste a lot of time thinking negative thoughts like, 'What if I don't do well?'

The nature of the mind is to run around in circles. Remember the monkey mind?

- Plan your work for each day. Organize yourself so that you have everything you need to study with attention.
- Practise pranayama such as anuloma viloma or bhramari pranayama (see Chapter 5).
- Make sure you're well rested and eating nourishing food.
- If you need help in any area, reach out to your teacher or parents.
- Write your affirmations or say them out loud to yourself in the mirror, 'I accept challenges as they come and I tackle them with confidence. I believe in myself. I've got this!'

Place your palms together in prayer pose at your chest. Hold the posture for 20 counts. Relax. Now complete the cycle by balancing on the other leg for the same amount of time. Observe how the mind feels now. BENEFIT: The practice of dharana means 'one-pointed focus'.

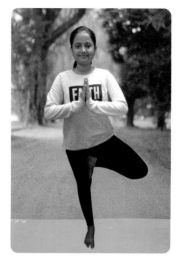

Vrikshasana

Have you noticed how we need to focus, especially when we don't like something very much? We focus single-mindedly while playing a video game or watching our favourite web series. However, there are times when we have to do things we don't like, for example, finish a boring chapter for an exam or complete a pending task. To complete the not-so-fun things, we need extra attention. We can improve the quality of focus and levels of concentration by practising Vrikshasana, or the tree pose.

When we consciously activate both sides of the brain, logical and creative, we find that the mind has more clarity through the day and enough energy to work, play and do things that need to be done.

Sitali

TECHNIQUE: Begin by taking in a deep breath through the nose and exhale fully through the mouth. Now make a tube with your tongue and let the tip

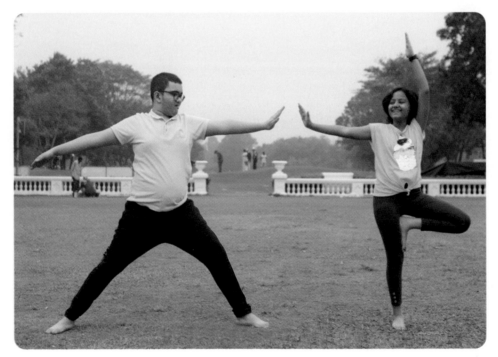

The dance of the left and right brain: living life in balance

peek out of the mouth. Breathe in through the mouth, feel your lungs fill with cool air and then exhale through the nose, slowly and steadily.

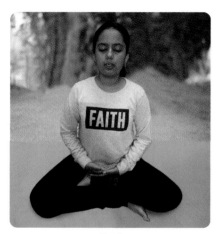
Sitali

BENEFIT: Sitali cools the stomach and invigorates the liver and spleen. It is like natural air conditioning for your internal organs and keeps the mind cool. If you feel tired after a long day at school or even angry at someone, this is the pranayama to try.

PIZZA SANDWICH

INGREDIENTS
- brown bread – 2 slices
- grated cheese – to taste
- tomatoes, onions, capsicums, lettuce – finely chopped
- salt, pepper – to taste
- homemade ketchup (see recipe in this chapter)

HOW TO MAKE IT
Grill slices of brown bread in the oven for 3 minutes. Spread homemade ketchup on one slice. Place the lettuce, tomatoes, onions, capsicum on the slice and sprinkle loads of cheese. Add salt and pepper. Cover with the other slice and get ready to munch!

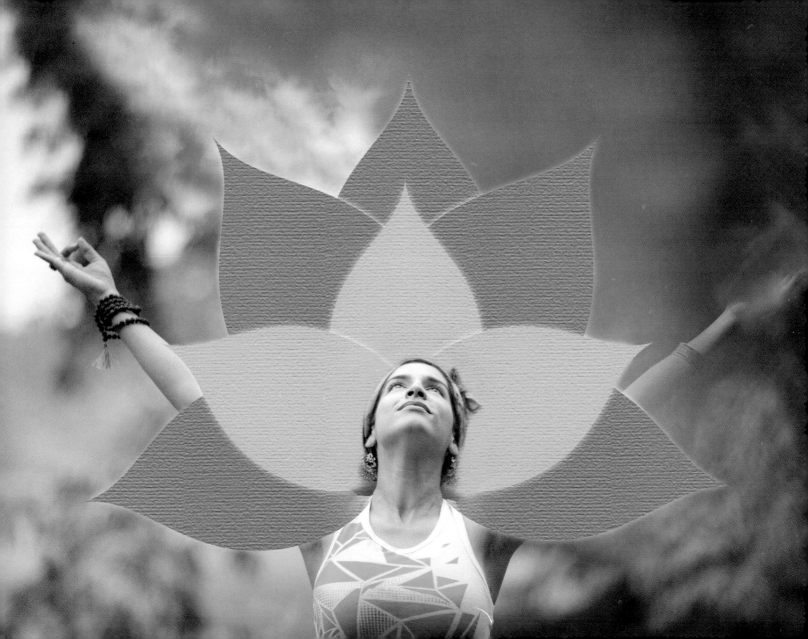

8

Loving the Cosmic You!

Every person, place, and thing on this planet is interconnected with love. I am at home in the universe.

LOUISE HAY
author

Our whole lives we have been told who we are. We have a name and an identity. We belong to a family, community, religion, gender, political affiliation, segment of society, demographic – and the list goes on.

We have often felt that we are more than any of these tags, yet we have let that feeling of enquiry pass and then continued to associate with the image that the outside world has built of us.

Close your eyes and observe the thoughts crossing your mind. Then ask yourself: who is this being, this strange person within me who is watching all my thoughts? Who am I?

It is true that we are more than what we can see. Made from elements into matter infused with life, we are more than skin and bones, more than our thoughts and more than the circumstances in our lives.

We must take time to appreciate what we have around us – the small externalities, the wonderful people in our lives, the efficiently functioning body that we have, the gift of our senses and, yes, even the daily challenges that make us stronger and braver.

Make it at home!

COCONUT BARFI

INGREDIENTS
- grated coconut – 2 cups
- brown sugar – 1 cup
- fresh cream – half cup
- green cardamom powder – 1 tsp

HOW TO MAKE IT
Heat a pan. Put in the coconut, cream and cardamom. Stir the mixture for 5–7 minutes. Add the sugar. Let the mixture turn slightly golden. Spread the mixture on a sheet and flatten it with a spoon. Allow it to cool. Cut into squares.

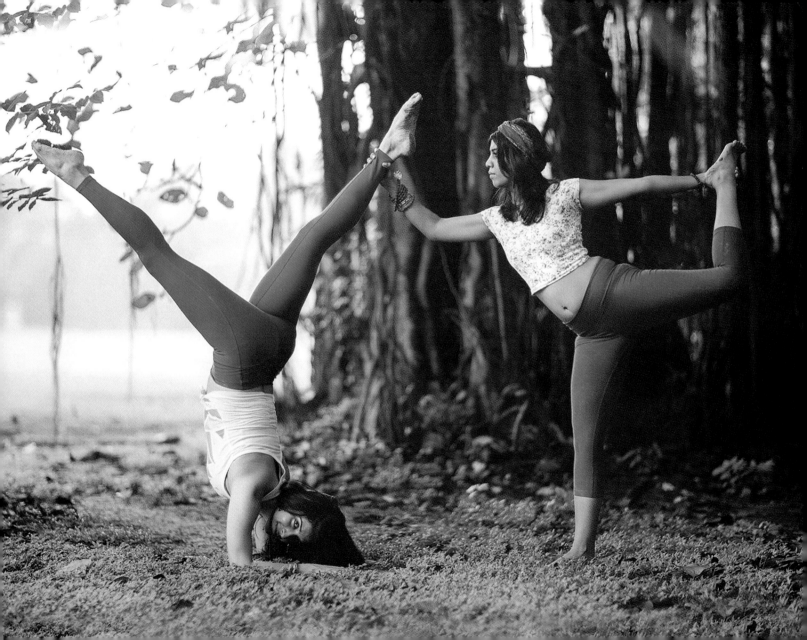

MOTHER NATURE

I got my period for the first time and stained my clothes. I was so embarrassed. I thought I was going to die.

Periods are a natural part of growing up. It is the body telling you that it is functioning as it should, that you are growing from a girl into a young lady.

- Staining your clothes, especially in blood, can seem frightening but if you've got truly cool friends they will know that it's okay and they will help you change. It is nothing to be ashamed of.
- Choose an environmentally friendly brand of sanitary pads that keeps your carbon footprint low.
- After you get your period, understand how your feelings and moods change. Talk to your close friends, or an adult you trust, about this experience. Educate yourself about the process.

Many of us begin to appreciate the things we have only when we don't have them anymore. Maybe being quarantined at home during the coronavirus pandemic made you realize how much you love going to school, or maybe you appreciate the meals cooked by your mother after being away for some time. When you realize how beautiful things were, and are, you begin to look at people and situations differently. You become grateful for the little things that make life worthwhile. When a friend saves a piece of that delicious chocolate for you, you thank them all the more, and maybe do something in return.

There comes a time in every life when each day seems difficult – sometimes even unbearable. Sometimes, these phases prove life changing. Even if they are not, it is important to remember that, just as fun is momentary, bad times too will pass.

Once we emerge from such times and look back, we find that we are not only stronger but better equipped to survive any future challenges. We managed to cross over. We got through. This is when we have to acknowledge that something inside us is constant. This is the *self*. From babyhood to adulthood, there is something inside us that doesn't change, even though we continually change on the outside. This 'self' is our hero. We are the heroes of our own lives.

No one can cross a turbulent ocean but ourself. The journey of our lives is to uncover the 'self'; the strongest, most permanent part of us; the beautiful, unchanging self that never leaves, no matter how old our body grows.

To love yourself is to love the most powerful force in the universe. You are the highest force of energy and you can channel it with the simple force of love. When you can love yourself, you will start a chain of love linking you to every person in your life. Sounds good, right?

> I love myself. The quietest, simplest, most powerful revolution ever.
> NAYYIRAH WAHEED, poet

More Than I Am

More than I,
And more than you,
We are more than just us two.
We're more than this body,
We are more than this face,
The world is our family,
The world is our space.
We have a heart,
So let it shine,
Open up,
And feel alive.
Let inner revolution be your song,
With love so soft and a mind so strong,
We simply cannot go wrong.
The world is our family,
The world is our place.
Let's stretch our arms,
And reach out with grace.
Those who await us,
Our smile, our love, our presence in this maze.
Vasudevakutumbakam – one world family,
The destination is one, but many are the ways.

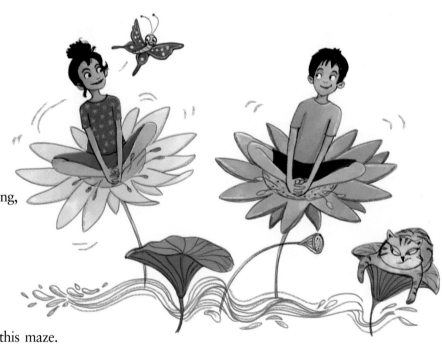

21-Day Sankalpa

PLEDGE

I recognize that I am made up of the mysterious elements of the universe and I am more than I can understand.

I, ... (name), undertake this 21-day sankalpa to become MORE THAN I AM.

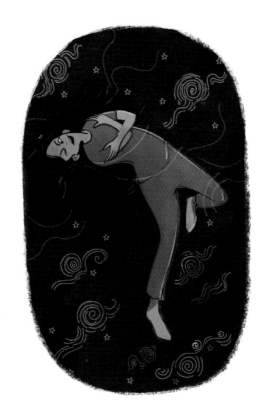

It has been said that it takes a minimum of 21 days to form a habit and that means that we have to practise any one action or skill for 21 days before it starts becoming a part of us. Sankalpa is a promise or an intention that we set for ourselves.

21 days = 3 weeks * 7 days per week

Each day = activity + abhyasa (practice) + meal

	ACTIVITY	ABHYASA	MEAL
DAY 1	Set an intention for yourself. Whatever you want to achieve, write it down on a piece of paper and hide it in your room.	Warm up and do one full round of suryanamaskar.	Add some violet-coloured foods to your meal – purple cabbage, onions, brinjal, beetroot, etc.
DAY 2	Practise self love by looking into the mirror and talking out loud to yourself about all the things you love about YOU. Be descriptive. Don't be shy.	Warm up and do two full rounds of suryanamaskar.	Snack on some nuts and seeds – walnuts, cashews, lotus seeds (makhana) – or raisins.
DAY 3	Do one good deed. Go up to a classmate or a junior and help them. It costs nothing to be good to others.	Warm up and do three full rounds of suryanamaskar.	Drink two full glasses of lukewarm water on an empty stomach before you start your day.

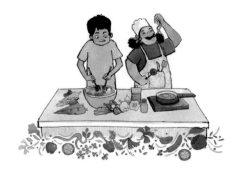

	ACTIVITY	ABHYASA	MEAL
DAY 4	Review all your previous homework and finish it even before your parents can tell you to do so. Surprise them by spending some quality time with them before bedtime. Sing them a song or discuss your day. Give them a BIG HUG.	Warm up and do four full rounds of suryanamaskar.	Some green foods are a must! Spinach, lady's finger and gourds are our best friends.
DAY 5	Spend five minutes staring out of your window at the sky. Set a timer. Feels good, doesn't it?	Warm up and do five full rounds of suryanamaskar.	Orange and yellow fruits and vegetables such as yellow peppers, carrots, pumpkin and others, work on building our immunity.

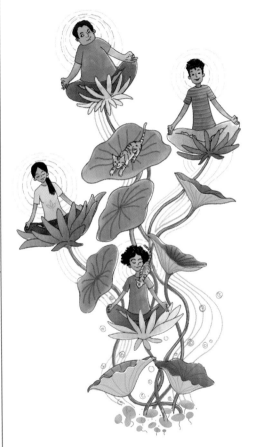

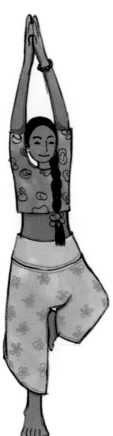

	ACTIVITY	ABHYASA	MEAL
DAY 6	Teach one family member a pranayama – bhastrika.	Warm up and do six full rounds of suryanamaskar.	Have khichdi or idli and sambar – the simplest possible meal. Full of protein, these rice and-pulses staples make us strong.
DAY 7	Consciously forgive someone who would have otherwise made you angry. Let nothing take away your smile.	Warm up and do seven full rounds of suryanamaskar.	Make a yogurt smoothie with a seasonal fruit of your choice.
DAY 8	Write down ten things you are grateful for in life.	Warm up and do eight full rounds of suryanamaskar.	Add a dash of red to your meal – apples, red bell peppers, red/brown rice. Make sure you clean the fruits/vegetables/grains well before cooking.

	ACTIVITY	ABHYASA	MEAL
DAY 9	Come up with one crazy idea that you think can change the world.	Warm up and do nine full rounds of suryanamaskar.	Eat your favourite meal.
DAY 10	Try and sit up straight the whole day. No slouching!	Warm up and do ten full rounds of suryanamaskar.	Plan a simple meal for your family that has different-coloured vegetables along with a little carbohydrate and proteins.
DAY 11	Watch a movie that always makes you laugh. Watch it with a friend.	Warm up and do eleven full rounds of suryanamaskar.	Try a bowl of mixed fruit salad for lunch.
DAY 12	Make a healthy snack for your parents.	Warm up and do twelve full rounds of suryanamaskar.	Snack on something healthy between meals – a piece of fruit, a juice or a homemade cookie.

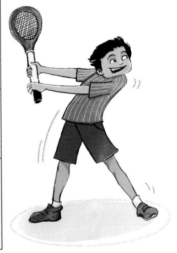

	ACTIVITY	ABHYASA	MEAL
DAY 13	Spend some time with your grandparents without getting impatient.	Warm up and do thirteen full rounds of suryanamaskar.	Have sweet potato chips and homemade ketchup as your evening snack.
DAY 14	Spend one whole day without your phone and social media.	Warm up and do fourteen full rounds of suryanamaskar.	Have soup for dinner.
DAY 15	Walk barefoot on the grass.	Warm up and do fifteen full rounds of suryanamaskar.	Drink some lukewarm water with a pinch of cinnamon and honey on an empty stomach.
DAY 16	Find five things in your kitchen that you think can be recycled.	Warm up and do sixteen full rounds of suryanamaskar.	Add some yogurt to your meal.

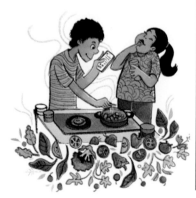

	ACTIVITY	ABHYASA	MEAL
DAY 17	Be a good listener. Sometimes all another person needs is a listening ear.	Warm up and do seventeen full rounds of suryanamaskar.	Snack on a big homemade burger to keep you happy.
DAY 18	What defines you? Create a picture by drawing, sketching or colouring a design that reflects you as a person.	Warm up and do eighteen full rounds of suryanamaskar.	Add a pinch each of black pepper and turmeric to a glass of milk and drink it before going to bed.
DAY 19	Wake up early and go for a morning walk.	Warm up and do nineteen full rounds of suryanamaskar.	Drink a glass of water with lemon, while standing, after lunch.

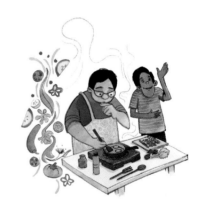

	ACTIVITY	ABHYASA	MEAL
DAY 20	Play an instrument even if you don't know how to.	Warm up and do twenty full rounds of suryanamaskar.	Eat a vegetable you don't like but know is good for you.
DAY 21	Say a prayer. Look back and absorb how much you've learnt in the last 21 days. Find the piece of paper you hid on the very first day and look at the intention you began with. Feel the gratitude.	Warm up and do twenty-one full rounds of suryanamaskar.	Make a salad. Add some cucumber and carrots with a dash of lime.

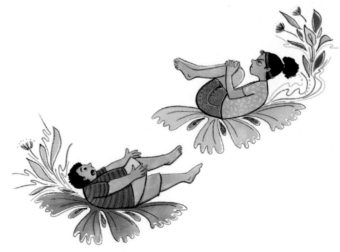

ABHYASA

routine of the day (asana and pranayama)

Abhyasa means a daily practice that we do consistently to bring inner strength and calm. Start with a warm-up to activate the muscles. Follow it up with more challenging postures to build flexibility and endurance.

STEP 1 – Warm up

1. Jumping jacks
2. Spot jogging
3. Standing twist
4. Neck rotation
5. Shoulder rotation
6. Arm rotation
7. Hip rotation
8. Knee rotation
9. Ankle rotation

Do rotations first in the clockwise direction and then in the anti-clockwise direction – ten times in each direction.

STEP 2

10. Asanas to strengthen and energize (Chapter 6)
11. Pranayamas and mudras – anuloma viloma/nadi shodhana, bhramari, merudanda (Chapter 5)
12. Suryanamaskar (Chapter 4) each day + 1 = total 21 days = 21 rounds (both legs)
13. Meditate for five minutes (Chapter 5).

Glossary

AGYA CHAKRA: energy vortex between the eyebrows

ANAHATA CHAKRA: energy vortex at the heart centre

APANAVAYU: energy that circulates downwards

ASANA: yoga postures or various scientific shapes that the body forms to enhance health and improve strength as mentioned in ancient texts like the *Yoga Sutras of Patanjali* and *Hatha Yoga Pradipika*.

CHAKRA: vortices or whirlpools of energy that feed the nadis or energy channels. There are seven types of chakras: sahasrara chakra, agya chakra, vishuddhi chakra, anahata chakra, manipura chakra, swadhistana chakra, mooladhara chakra.

EK TATTVA ABHYASA: one-pointed practice, or practising one thing can bring you perfection and overcome any obstacle

MANIPURA CHAKRA: energy vortex at the navel

MOOLADHARA CHAKRA: energy vortex four fingers above the mooladhara/spine

NADIS: invisible energy channels in the body through which prana passes

OJAS: glow or vitality. According to the Rasashastra (the branch of Ayurveda that specializes in chemicals, herbs, minerals and metals), Ojas is enhanced by eating the right food and living the right lifestyle.

PRANA: the life force that sustains us

PRANAVAYU: energy that circulates upwards (NOTE: Pranavayu is a subset of prana. Prana and pranavayu are not the same thing.)

SAHASRARA CHAKRA: energy vortex on the top of the head

SAMANAVAYU: energy that circulates around the navel, working on digestion and assimilation

SAMATVAM YOGA UCCHYATE: the practice of yoga gives you a balanced and equanimous body and mental state, even when life has ups and downs.

SUSHUMNA: central energy channel corresponding with the spine

SWADHISTANA CHAKRA: energy vortex four inches below the navel

UDANAVAYU: energy that circulates around the throat and head and works on the mental faculties

VAYUS: literally means 'wind' and, within the body, refers to an energetic force that controls bodily functions and activities. There are five types of vayus: pranavayu, apanavayu, samanavayu, udanavayu and vyanavayu.

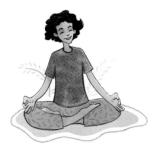

VISHUDDHI CHAKRA: energy vortex in the throat region

VYANAVAYU: energy that works on the body's circulation

Further Reading

1. *Yoga Sutras of Patanjali*
2. *Asana, Pranayama, Mudra, Bandha* by Swami Satyananda Saraswati
3. *Light on Yoga* by B.K.S. Iyengar
4. *The Bhagwad Gita*
5. *Hatha Yoga Pradipika* by Svātmārāma
6. *Autobiography of a Yogi* by Paramhansa Yogananda
7. *Yoga Anatomy* by Leslie Kaminoff

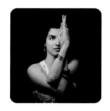

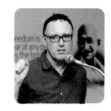

Varuna Shunglu is an international yoga teacher, wellness entrepreneur and lawyer. She has a MSc in Yogic Sciences and is certified by Yoga Alliance International. Varuna has written for publications such as *The Telegraph*, *Asia Spa*, *Men's Health* and the *Business Standard*.

Ken Spillman is a professional author and speaker. He has written more than 90 books, published in dozens of languages worldwide.

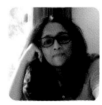

Suvidha Mistry has illustrated for various publishing houses in India. Her book cover for *The Naughty Bear* written by Paro Anand, was awarded by 'Publishing Next' in 2019. She's been honoured by the Association of Writers and Illustrators for Children and has participated in the Nambook010, International Children's Book Festival, Korea 2010. Her works have been exhibited in Korea and Bratislava.